the
BEESWAX
WORKSHOP

How to Make Your Own Natural Candles, Cosmetics, Cleaners, Soaps, Healing Balms and More

CHRIS DALZIEL

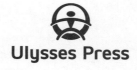

Ulysses Press

Published in the United States by:
Ulysses Press
P.O. Box 3440
Berkeley, CA 94703
www.ulyssespress.com

ISBN: 978-1-61243-648-7
Library of Congress Catalog Number 2016950667

Printed in the United States by United Graphics Inc.
10 9 8 7 6 5 4 3 2 1

Acquisitions editor: Bridget Thoreson
Project manager: Casie Vogel
Managing editor: Claire Chun
Editor: Renee Rutledge
Proofreader: Shayna Keyles
Indexer: Sayre Van Young
Cover design: Malea Clark-Nicholson
Cover photo: © Eskymaks/shutterstock.com
Interior design: what!design @ whatweb.com
Interior photos: © Chris Dalziel except pages 1, 10 © Angi Schneider/
    SchneiderPeeps.com, page 7 © Connie Meyers, and pages 180, 298 ©
    Elliot Teskey

Distributed by Publishers Group West

To my one for all time, Robin, I5005EU

CONTENTS

FOREWORD

I grew up in a traditional farm family. And by traditional, I mean there was none of that hippie organic stuff. It was the '70s, and while some people were embracing new-fangled supermarket products like yogurt and granola, my folks were having none of that.

Our family farm did sell honey from a local beekeeper, though. With white table sugar so readily available and inexpensive, natural honey was still a stretch for my mom's table, but she couldn't really quibble with it. One summer day the beekeeper brought a special gift of golden yellow bee pollen for us, raving about the health benefits of this bee by-product. My mom secretly rolled her eyes.

People have been using bee pollen as a superfood for thousands of years and it's touted as a source of eternal youth. As it fell out of favor, though, it became a bit of an oddity. These days we embrace scientifically developed cosmetics and supplements that promise to reduce aging, improve energy, and boost vitality. And we've been buying into it for decades.

As I was writing this, that beekeeper's name came to me. It's been 30 years or more since I've seen him, but a quick Internet search brought up his photo. Let me tell you. That bee pollen (and arguably, his "alternative" lifestyle that embraced bee pollen) has done wonders for his aging process. He doesn't look a day older than he did all those years ago.

Beeswax has followed a trajectory similar to that of bee pollen. Once commonly used in households, this naturally-derived product has

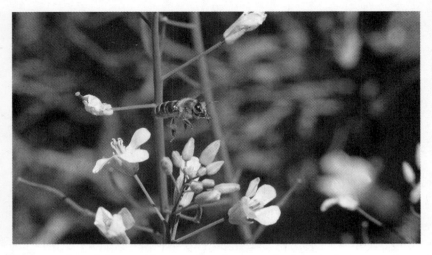

been replaced by modern technology and chemical concoctions created in a laboratory.

Take candles, for instance. Most candles on the market these days are made of petroleum-based paraffin and scented with artificial fragrances created in a laboratory. The federal government has established regulations to ensure that the volatile organic compounds emitted from these candles are at a "safe" level. A beeswax candle, on the other hand, is made of beeswax, pure and simple.

It's heartening for me to see that many people are beginning to turn to more natural alternatives. Choosing to use products with simpler, gentler ingredients reduces exposure to toxic compounds in the household, and prevents those compounds from making their way into our environment. With modern ingredients like triclosan and microbeads being removed from products almost as quickly as they are added due to safety and environmental concerns, it certainly seems sensible to turn to less caustic options.

Switching to less toxic products in the home is the first step on a path toward creating a healthier environment for family and friends. Making your own common household and beauty products at home takes it a step further. Not only do handmade products remove toxins and harsh chemicals from the environment, but they reduce the amount of disposable packaging heading to the landfill, as well.

The projects and homemade products included in this book are a great starting point for consumers who are ready to try something different. Chris Dalziel offers up a huge collection of small-batch recipes that are easy enough for anyone to tackle. If you can follow instructions, you can make the products included here in less than an hour. That's probably less time than it would take you to run to the store!

From making body products like ointments, salves, cosmetics, and lotions to creating grafting wax for the garden or waterproofing shoes or caring for leather, there's something here for everyone. Replacing your household standbys with a less toxic option is something that you can easily do, one product at a time, as you begin your journey to a more self-reliant lifestyle.

—Kris Bordessa

Attainable Sustainable
Make your own. Grow your own. OWN your life.
http://candles.org/faqs

INTRODUCTION

Beeswax is woven into my story. It pleasantly scents my home, gives me something useful to make for the craft markets, textures and preserves my herbal remedies, waterproofs my garden equipment, and lights my Friday nights with its sweet, golden light.

It began when my husband, two sons, and I stopped at an open-air, agritourism market because we saw the sign "Planet Bee" on the highway. It was impromptu. The boys were hot and restless. We all needed a break from driving. The sign promised ice cream and bathrooms.

At Planet Bee, a honey farm and shop in British Columbia's Okanagan Valley, we watched as a beekeeper, dressed in a short-sleeve white

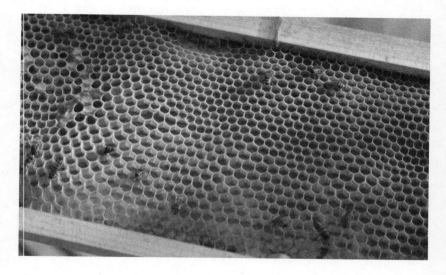

shirt without any other protective clothing, pulled a frame covered in bees out of a wooden box. They flew around him on stage and crawled on his bare hands as he explained to the audience the gentle nature of bees. We didn't need to be afraid of them. He asked us not to run from them and not to swat at them if any accidentally landed on us during the demonstration. He said if a bee stung us, it would release a pheromone that would tell the other bees to come and sting us, too. However, the bees did not want to sting.

He moved slowly, deliberately, as he told us about how the bees pollinated the Okanagan fruit crop. Without the bees there would be no peaches, apples, apricots, or cherries. My youngest son, just six, watched with toothless rapture. The nine year old was eager to try the honey samples.

After the show we wandered around the store. I found a replica colonial tin mold for making taper candles. It was a decor piece, not actually meant to be used as a mold. There was no wax or wicks on the market shelves, and no books on how to make candles. I asked the girl behind the counter if they had any beeswax. She shrugged and left to get the beekeeper. He told me he only had big, 30-pound blocks of beeswax. One cost $150, but he'd let me have it for $130 if I took the whole block. "Sure," I said.

He led me to a back room. The golden beeswax was like a wheel of cheese, from which I learned how to slice off pieces of wax on the spot using an ax. After that, I was on my own with a tin candle mold and a 30-pound stash of beeswax. It was 1991.

By that November I had made my first beeswax candles, after several failures. At Christmas, everyone over nineteen received beeswax candles and homemade soap. Beeswax and I were officially "in a relationship."

Twenty-five years later, I'm buying 5 pounds of beeswax annually from a local beekeeper. The price has risen about 40 percent in that time. I now use it for many more things around our home and garden. In this book I share my personal recipes for everything from candles to cosmetics, cleaning supplies to art supplies, and even useful preparations for the household and for sports activities.

Beeswax replaces many of the toxic, petroleum-based products you may now be using. It is useful as a protectant, lubricant, and stabilizer. It can be either solid or malleable depending on the temperature. It improves the texture of other products. In health preparations and cosmetics, beeswax is a humectant and moisturizer. It is antimicrobial and rich in vitamin A, with trace amounts of pollen and propolis, the tree resins collected by honeybees. When it burns as a candle, beeswax combats indoor air pollution by releasing negative ions into the air, refreshing it with its sweet honey scent.

Chapter 1
MIRACULOUS BEESWAX

There is one masterpiece, the hexagonal cell, which touches perfection. No living creature, not even man, has achieved, in the center of his sphere, what the bee has achieved in her own: and were someone from another world to descend and ask of the earth the most perfect creation of the logic of life, we should needs have to offer the humble comb of honey.

—Maurice Maeterlinck, *The Life of the Bee* (1924)

The Honeybee

Several different kinds of bees, including bumblebees, produce a waxy substance, but beeswax, as we know it, is produced by the western honeybee *(Apis mellifera)* to enclose their brood and their winter food. The wax is made by four pairs of wax glands on the abdomens of 12-day-old daughter bees. These wax glands function efficiently for just five days. During this time, the wax glands exude thin wax scales that are manipulated by the bees to build the hexagon-shaped cells that make up the honeycomb.

The honeycomb is a feat of miraculous engineering. When left to design their own hive structure, honeybees will fit each hexagon tightly with the other hexagons in a pattern that forms a womb-like structure. The cells of the hive are used both for brood cells and

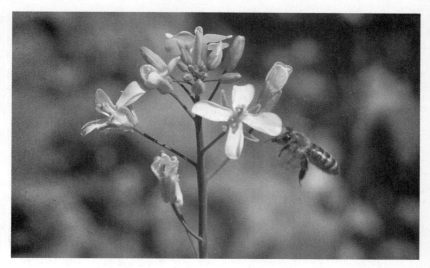

for honey storage. During wax production, the daughter bees must consume 6 to 8 pounds of honey to produce 1 pound of wax. That 1 pound of wax will hold 22 pounds of honey efficiently.

The average yield of honey and wax is dependent on a lot of factors, including the size of the colony, available forage, and the ancestry of the honeybees. A single colony can produce 300 pounds of honey and 15 pounds of wax in a single season. However, much of that is used by the bees themselves to raise their brood and survive the winter. In a good year, the beekeeper may be able to harvest 30 to 80 pounds of honey and just 1 or 2 pounds of wax from one colony. In a poor year, the bees need all their honey to survive the winter.

How Do Bees Make Beeswax?

While some people speak of the hive as if it is a political entity, I like to think of it as a family. Every bee is the son or daughter of the same mother, and each bee has a job to do. The male bees, or drones, have only one task: to mate with a queen bee and produce more daughters. The daughters carry on all the age-appropriate household duties, gaining more responsibilities as they mature.

The first job of a new daughter bee is to clean her room. If her brood cell isn't cleaned well enough, the mother bee sends her back to clean it again. Once her own brood cell is clean, she learns how to keep the hive clean and warm. By the time she is three days old, she is ready to babysit the older larvae in the hive. After she's mastered this job, she moves on to taking care of the youngest larvae, preparing their food, and feeding them.

By the time she's twelve days old, she is producing wax scales, building comb, carrying food, storing food for winter, and making the medicine needed by the other bees to keep them healthy and strong. When these young daughters are 18 to 20 days old, they are promoted to guard status. Their job is to protect the hive from intruders. They are ready to give up their lives for the protection of their family. After just three days as guards, they graduate to full worker bee status. From this point on, these daughters will leave the hive at dawn to forage for food for the colony, returning several times a day with nectar and pollen.

Bees aren't union workers with only one job, though. If at any time the clan requires a job done and there are not sufficient bees of the right age to do it, the older daughters pick up the slack to help the colony survive, just like in a family. Foraging bees are capable of making wax in their atrophied wax glands. If necessary, these older daughters can make food and medicine, keep the hive temperature stable, seal the drafts, and clean.

Colony Collapse Disorder

You've probably heard of colony collapse disorder. Honey bee populations worldwide reached a critical low point in 2007, with entire colonies dying off during the winter of 2006–2007. As I write this, many countries are showing honeybees in recovery after 10 years of concentrated efforts to establish habitat and reduce pesticide use.

The key pesticides blamed for the decline in the western honeybee and wild bee populations are neonicotinoid pesticides. Neonicotinoid pesticides are used to treat the seeds of plants to protect against insect damage, which leads to crop loss. Neonicotinoid pesticides are systemic pesticides. When seeds are treated with neonicotinoids, every cell of the growing plant is pesticide laden, including the pollen and nectar. When bees forage these plants, individual bees are poisoned. These bees bring the nectar from these plants back to the hive. Many of these forager bees die from exposure to neonicotinoids.

In some cases, the hive is able to recover from the devastating loss of forager bees by hatching more female worker bees. However, the neonicotinoid-laced nectar is stored in the colony as honey and is consumed by the colony during the winter months, leading to colony collapse disorder. Further, neonicotinoids harm the reproductive capacity of male bees, reducing the lifespan of drones and damaging sperm viability. This further weakens bee colonies.

The EU placed a ban on neonicotinoid use in 2013. Research is ongoing in Europe.

In the United States, the EPA and the Department of Agriculture are researching the connection between bee deaths and neonicotinoid use. However, their results will not be released until 2018. In 2016, Maryland and Connecticut became the first states to ban consumer use of neonicotinoids. Agricultural, horticultural, and veterinary use of the pesticides is still permitted.

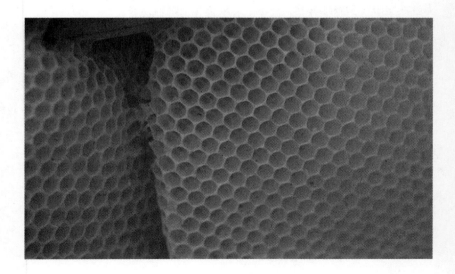

What Can You Do?

There are a few things you can do to help the bees.

Plant nectar-producing plants, with the bees in mind. One of the factors in the decline of pollinators is the loss of habitat to development. As more people consciously plant masses of flowering, nectar-producing plants that bloom over a long season, the bees will have more opportunities to make the nectar and the medicine that they need to strengthen the colony.

Bees forage one kind of plant at a time. If the bees are foraging kale plants, they will continue foraging kale and ignore other flowers that are open nearby. By planting masses of one type of flower, the bees have more opportunities to feed and to gather.

Grow an organic garden. By growing food organically, you will avoid the use of pesticides. This gives the bees a safe place to forage. It also increases awareness of the pollinators and their health. Gardeners need pollinators.

Adopt a beehive. Last summer I saw beekeeping equipment for the first time in a local Home Hardware store. There were beehives, protective clothing, smokers, and books on beekeeping for sale. Before the Industrial Revolution, keeping bees was a normal activity for gardeners. Gardeners kept a hive or two in the back garden to supply honey and wax, and to pollinate the fruit trees. Today, even city dwellers are adopting beehives and learning about honeybee husbandry. The information that beginning beekeepers need is more accessible than it used to be. Talk to a local beekeeper about adopting a hive with bees that are already acclimatized to your local area.

Buy local honey and wax. Not everyone can adopt a beehive. If you can't, buy local honey and wax directly from the beekeeper. This helps your local economy. It lets the beekeeper know that there is a market for her inventory. It encourages her to keep going.

Beeswax Basics

There are different kinds and qualities of wax. Freshly made beeswax is white. Golden beeswax gets its color from the pollen and honey stored in the wax comb. Here's more on the various kinds of wax you might encounter:

Brood wax. This is a very dark wax melted from comb that was previously used to hold bee larvae. Some beekeepers reuse the same wax foundation over and over in order to save the bees' energy and honey. When bees have to build honeycomb before they can lay eggs, it takes longer to get the colony growing in the spring. But when the wax is reused over and over, it becomes dark with propolis, honey, and bee gunk. This older wax is the lowest quality. You'll need to render it by melting it down with a bit of water to let the impurities sink out of the wax before you can use it for the recipes in this book. There will be a lot of waste.

Honeycomb with the honey still in it is sometimes sold in the market. The wax comb is meant to be eaten with the honey as a delicacy. In a jar of honey with the comb, the comb represents a very small portion of the jar. To separate the wax from the honey, cut the comb with a knife to open all the honey cells. Strain the honey from the comb. Then, render the wax in a large quantity of water. The impurities, the honey, and the propolis will drop to the bottom of the pan. The wax will float on top and can be skimmed off.

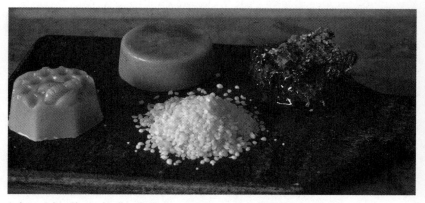

Left to right: Cleaned yellow beeswax, capping wax, pastilles, honeycomb

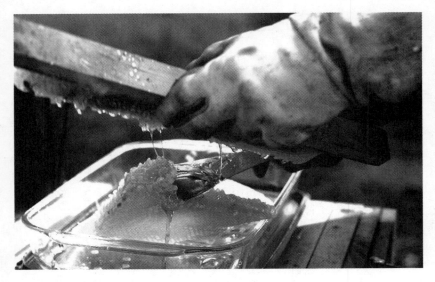

Capping wax. This is the most common wax you'll encounter. It is the first rendered wax from the beekeeper. Capping wax should be rendered one more time, without water, before you use it to make candles, cosmetics, or apothecary items. It is golden wax, but may have a trace amount of residual honey, bee parts, or dirt embedded in the wax. I find that melting a block of capping wax in my wax pot and keeping it warm for an hour to let the junk settle allows me to separate the cleaned yellow wax from the gunk at the bottom of the container. Just pour off the top layer of yellow wax into silicone molds, and pour off the darker, gunky wax into its own mold and save it for recipes that call for waste wax.

Cleaned yellow beeswax. This is cosmetic-grade beeswax, cleaned of all residual honey, bee parts, and propolis. It's ready to use for any of the recipes in this book. This is the grade of wax you'll need for candlemaking. Expect to pay more for cleaned beeswax than you would for capping wax.

White filtered beeswax. This beeswax has been filtered of all honey and bee parts. It's been bleached either by exposure to UV light or by filtering through a carbon filter. This is the best grade of wax to use when making art supplies; colored wax will shift the colors, making them less bright. White beeswax often lacks the characteristic honey scent associated with 100 percent beeswax. Expect to pay more for white filtered beeswax than you would for cleaned yellow beeswax.

Working with Blocks of Wax

Large blocks of wax are difficult to work with. While the beekeeper suggested I chip off pieces of the wax "cheese" with an axe, this is neither a safe nor effective process. Solid wax is hard and doesn't give way to chipping without protest. If you must deal with a large block of wax, melt it in a pot over low heat.

Wax is flammable, though—it will spontaneously burst into flames at 400°F, the flash point of beeswax. You only need to get it between 140°F and 147°F, the point at which beeswax melts. It will discolor at 185°F. Using a double boiler to melt wax ensures that the temperature remains below the critical point. Even when using a double boiler, never leave a pot of melting wax unattended.

If you encounter a wax fire, do not throw water on it. Wax fires, like grease fires, will explode as water droplets evaporate when they hit the wax. This could send a rolling fireball into the air. Instead, smother a wax fire using sand, salt, a fire extinguisher, or a wool blanket.

Caution: Do not melt wax with young children or pets in the room. Keep pot handles turned to the back of the stove at all times so that children don't tip a pot of hot wax on themselves because they wanted to see what was in it. If you spill any on your skin, remove the wax immediately and run your skin under the cold water tap. Aloe vera gel will help cool a minor burn quickly. For more serious burns, consult your medical professional.

Blocks of beeswax weighing less than 3 pounds can be melted in a can placed inside a large pot, like a soup pot or pasta pot. Fill the large pot with water so that it comes at least halfway up the can. Simmer over medium heat. This is a makeshift double boiler.

I find it easier to melt larger blocks of wax in this way, using a tin can inside a large pot. Once beeswax blocks are fully melted, any impurities will drop out of the wax to the bottom of the can. I pour the cleaned, rendered wax into smaller 1-, 2-, and 4-ounce blocks. Silicone molds are easiest to use for this. Several sizes are available. See the Resource section on page 278 for sources of molds.

Ingredients with a higher melting point should be melted before adding beeswax to the recipe to avoid damaging the crystalline structure of beeswax with high heat. This chart lists the melting points for several waxes and resins.

MELTING POINTS OF WAXES AND RESINS

Bayberry	102°F to 120°F
Beeswax	140°F to 147°F
Paraffin	107°F to 147°F (depends on formulation)
Candelilla wax	149°F to 156°F
Pine rosin	176°F
Carnauba wax	183°F to 185°F
Damar resin	248°F

If you are using a hard plastic mold, spray it with food-grade silicone spray before filling it with beeswax. This saves a lot of frustration when you go to unmold it.

To use the blocks of wax for any of the recipes in this book, assume 1 tablespoon of beeswax weighs 12 grams. Weigh the block of wax on a kitchen scale to determine the volume.

Beeswax pastilles, or pellets, are sold in 1-pound packages. They are higher priced than blocks of beeswax. They don't require melting before you measure them, saving you time. They come in both yellow/beige beeswax and white beeswax. The colored beeswax has the sweet honey scent; white beeswax is odorless. To measure the beeswax pastilles, press the beeswax in your fingers and into the spoon, causing the wax to stick together and form a solid clump.

The recipes in this book are written using volume measurements. When working with solid blocks of beeswax, it's sometimes easier to measure beeswax by weight. Use this chart to convert your beeswax from weight measurement to volume measurement.

Volume in recipe	Weight in ounces	Weight in grams
1 teaspoon	.14 ounce	4 grams
1 tablespoon	.42 ounce	12 grams
2 tablespoons	.85 ounce	24 grams
3 tablespoons	1.27 ounces	36 grams
¼ cup	1.7 ounces	48 grams
½ cup	3.39 ounces	96 grams
¾ cup	5.08 ounces	144 grams
1 cup	6.77 ounces	192 grams

Cleaning Up Wax

Pliable, malleable, sticky, hard when cold—the characteristics of beeswax that make it desirable for making stuff are the same characteristics that make it hard to clean up. As I write this, there is a 3-inch circle of beeswax splattered on the floor beside my stove. It's collecting gritty dirt. By the time you read this, it will have been cleaned up, I promise.

Lay down newspaper or parchment paper in your work area to catch wax drips. It will make clean up easier. I use an old sheet as a drop sheet when I'm making dipped candles to avoid those splotches on the vinyl floor.

Spilled wax can be cleaned up off the floor or counters by applying ice cubes to the wax because beeswax becomes brittle at freezing temperatures. You'll be able to scrape the residual wax up with a blunt knife once it's been iced for a few minutes. Often, spilled wax will lift off smooth countertops, stove tops, and sinks without scraping.

When cleaning up the dishes after doing one of the projects in this book, wipe out the containers, spoons, and pots of residual wax with a paper towel. You can discard the towel in your compost bucket. Beeswax is biodegradable, as are all the ingredients in these recipes. Once the residual wax is removed, wash the dish in hot, soapy water.

Glass measuring cups can be immersed in the simmering water that you used for melting the beeswax. Avoid burning yourself when you do this. I usually let them get cool enough to pick them up without burning my hands. The wax inside them should still be soft, so it can be easily wiped off. Once the residual wax is wiped away, the glasses and tins clean easily with dishwashing liquid.

Wax is difficult to get out of metal pots, so you'll be happier if you have a pot that is reserved for melting beeswax. Garage sales and thrift stores are good places to find suitable pots. You might even luck out and find a double boiler for a cheap price.

Under no circumstance should you pour beeswax down the drain. Liquid beeswax will become solid in your plumbing pipes, necessitating a costly repair. Dishes that are thick with beeswax need to have the wax removed before washing. I keep a silicone mold just for pouring out leftover beeswax when I'm working with it. This keeps the melting pot clean and gives me smaller blocks of beeswax to work with when I want to make a project.

Paper towels or rags that are soaked in linseed oil or solvent, used for clean up, should be fully dried and then safely disposed of. They are a combustion hazard as long as they are wet.

Necessary Equipment

A few important pieces of equipment are needed for working with beeswax, no matter which recipe you want to make. Beeswax should be melted in a double boiler rather than in a pot directly on the stove top or over an open flame. Here are the three types of double boilers called for in the recipes.

Tin can double boiler. A double boiler can be created by placing a tin can in a larger pot. Fill the larger pot with a few inches of water, and simmer the water to create a double boiler. The heat will transfer from the simmering water to the can containing beeswax and the beeswax will melt. I use this kind of double boiler when the recipe has resins or shellac in it. Resins and shellac melt at higher temperatures than beeswax, and they are stickier and harder to clean up out of the melting pot. Tin cans don't need to be cleaned, and can be discarded after use. When I want you to use this kind of double boiler in the recipe, I'll say, "Create a double boiler using a tin can."

Glass measuring cup double boiler. For the cosmetic recipes in this book, I use a glass, heatproof measuring cup inside a saucepan. I use a canning jar ring in the bottom of the saucepan to hold the glass measuring cup off the bottom of the pan. Fill the pan with enough water so it comes halfway up the sides of the glass cup. Most recipes in this book can be made utilizing this kind of double boiler, and when I want you to use one, I'll say, "Create a double boiler using a glass measuring cup."

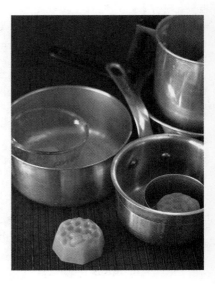

Deep wax pot double boiler. When melting wax for candles, you'll need a deeper wax pot. Specialized wax pots with built-in spouts and a heatproof handle make this job easier. They can be purchased for around $12 on Amazon. Alternatively, a 3-quart can, such as the kind that olive oil is sold in, works. Using pliers, pinch the rim on one side of the can to make a spout. Place the wax pot or can in a large pot with water that comes at least halfway up the side of the wax pot. This will allow you to melt the wax easily.

When you need to use this kind of double boiler in a recipe, I'll say, "Create a double boiler using a deep wax pot."

The Recipes

The projects in this book are more like craft projects than recipes. Nevertheless, I've written each one as if it were a recipe. I want you to feel that making any of these projects is more like playing in the kitchen than working in a laboratory. They are all within reach and doable. Those who have gone before us needed these same items in their homes and used beeswax to meet the need. It's only recently in human history that these items were manufactured under laboratory and factory conditions using synthetic wax.

These recipes are highly customizable. I introduce a variety of ingredients so that you can become familiar with their various properties. The key ingredients and the qualities they contribute to the recipes are described in detail in the Ingredient Guide on page 258. If you are allergic to nuts and the recipe calls for walnut oil, just flip to the section on Walnut Oil (page 272) to see which other oils contribute the same drying qualities, and you'll find a suitable substitute. Make all substitutions on a cup for cup, teaspoon for teaspoon basis unless otherwise noted. When you substitute an ingredient, the recipe will not be exactly the same, but it should still serve the same purpose. As you get to know the ingredients and how they behave in each formula, my hope is that you'll tweak each recipe to fit your own needs and lifestyle.

Should you go out with a shopping list and buy every single ingredient mentioned in the book? Some of the ingredients you'll already have on hand. Some are specialty items. I suggest you purchase items on an as-needed basis. It's more fun that way. As you build your supply cupboard, you'll figure out which ingredients you'll need over and over again and which ingredients you'll hardly use. See Resources on page 278 for a list of suppliers.

Some of the ingredients in these recipes can be found in nature. Some medicinal herbs and common weeds are growing in your neighborhood. If you decide to harvest them for the recipes in this book, make a positive identification in at least three ways if the plant is new to you. Use a field guide written for your area. Ask a friend experienced in foraging. Only when you are positive of the identification of the herb should you harvest it.

Herbs can be dried as soon as you harvest them by hanging them up in bundles and letting them air dry, out of direct sunlight. Once the herbs are fully dry, they can be stored in glass jars or infused in oil. They can be used in the recipes in this book in either state.

Is This Sustainable?

I'm often asked whether this do-it-yourself lifestyle is sustainable. That's like asking, can we all raise our own vegetables or fruit trees or clothing? Our ancestors did, so it's in the realm of possibility.

I don't think "Is this sustainable?" is the right question because it assumes the status quo is the best way. Instead we must ask, "What are we willing to change to make it work?"

As more and more people garden, plant nectar-producing flowers, and adopt bee families, there is a strong move toward positive change.

It begins with people valuing the honeybee and her products. We should not take as much as possible from the hive, but rather give the bee a resilient neighborhood to raise a family in. In this way, the bees can produce abundantly, with enough left over for us to share.

Chapter 2
BEESWAX
CANDLEMAKING

Good people are like candles; they burn
themselves up to give others light.

—Turkish proverb

For many people, candlemaking is a good introduction to working with beeswax. Beeswax is one of the most desirable waxes for candles. Beeswax candles are a healthy alternative to cheaper, petroleum-based candles. Paraffin candles are shown to negatively affect indoor air quality because of the chemical by-products in their soot. All paraffin candles produce soot. Beeswax candles burn cleanly, without soot.

Some people opt for vegetable waxes, like soy wax. Soy wax is made from hydrogenated soybean oil. It can go rancid in storage. Beeswax is stable in storage and will not deteriorate at normal room temperatures, even after thousands of years.

Beeswax candles are easy to make at home. From candles made from beeswax sheets to novelty molded candles, beeswax is versatile and easy to use. Beeswax releases a sweet honey scent as it burns, which becomes more pronounced when the candle flame is extinguished. Essential oil scents can be added to beeswax candles to offer ambiance and natural fragrance.

The quality of your beeswax can affect the success of your candles. Beeswax from local sources may need to be rendered a second time (see Capping Wax on page 10) before being used for candles. While you don't need white filtered wax for candle making, your wax should be free of residual honey and insect parts.

Never Leave a Burning Candle Unattended

Attending a burning candle is being in the same room, awake, with your eyes open. I learned this the hard way on a day I had an intimate group of people over for a bible study. There was a strange flickering glow coming from the dining room. I could see it from where I sat in the living room.

I got up discreetly to investigate the glow. The candles I had placed on the dining room table had dripped and burned down to the candle-holders. The flame, accelerated by a ceiling fan, was 2 feet high, the wooden candleholders acting like secondary wicks, fueled by a pool of melted wax on the table. I grabbed a tablecloth from a drawer and smothered the flame while simultaneously sweeping the whole mess into the tablecloth and out onto the back lawn. Then I quietly returned to my seat in the bible study. My guests never knew how close we had come to disaster.

Lesson learned: never leave a burning candle unattended. Tea lights are safer than tapers or votives in a situation like this. They are self-contained in a flameproof holder and will self-extinguish.

Wellness Benefits of Beeswax Candles

Beeswax emits negative ions when it burns. Negative ions clean the air of odors and bacteria. Falling water, like waterfalls, rain, and snow, also gives off negative ions. That smell after a spring rain is the negative ions doing their job. In a similar way, beeswax candles clean the indoor air.

Beeswax candles do not release the toxic chemicals that occur in paraffin candle soot. However, to ensure a clean burn, a properly sized wick should be used in each candle.

Types of Candles

There are a few common types of candles that you might make at home. Each kind has a different use.

Tea light. Tea light candles are small 1-inch wax candles with an integrated cup that also serves as a candle holder. Tea light candles are used as heat sources under teapots, as well as lighting for festive occasions. They are very safe to use because they are self-contained and their flame self-extinguishes when the wax pool is consumed in the candle flame. A beeswax tea light candle will burn for 4 hours.

Votive. Votive candles are small candles that must be put in a special votive holder to burn. The wick is sized so that the votive candle is fully melted and consumed in the flame. The votive holder catches the melting wax and prevents it from pooling. They have traditionally been used as symbols of prayer and devotion in religious ritual. Votive candles burn for 15 to 23 hours, depending on the height of the candle.

Taper. Taper candles are slender and tall candles that are typical of the kinds of candles used during formal occasions. Tapers are usually 8 to 9 inches tall and ¾ to ⅞ inch diameter at the base, tapering gradually along the length to a ½-inch diameter at the top of the candle. Tapers are sized to fit standard candle holders. Tapers generally burn for 1¼ hours per inch of candle height.

Pillar. Pillar candles vary in diameter and height but are larger than tea-light and votive candles. Pillar candles are decorative and have a long burn time. The flame generally burns down the center of the candle, leaving a thin layer of wax on the sides of the candle intact. This outer layer of wax glows warmly as the wick burns inside the pillar. Pillar candles are commonly made in a mold. These Pillar candles vary in burn time, depending on the diameter of the candle and the size of the wick.

Jar candles. Jar candles are pillar candles that remain in their mold, rather than being removed. They are very safe because the wax and the flame are contained in jar. These candles are as decorative as the jar that is used to hold the wax. Jar candles are often used as emergency candles. They vary in burn time, depending on the diameter of the jar and the size of the wick.

Candle Wicking

The wick is the most important part of the candle. The size of the wick and the composition of the wax determine the rate of burn as well as the cleanness of the burn. Ideally, all the wax in a candle should be liquefied by the flame and pulled into the wick by capillary action, being fully consumed by the flame. To achieve this, the wick must be big enough to draw up the liquid wax into the flame before it drips down the side of the candle, yet the wick should be small enough not to melt such a large pool of wax that the flame cannot consume it, allowing the wick to drown in the pool of wax.

The wick is a braided bundle of cotton, linen, or hemp thread that has been mordanted in a salt solution to inhibit burning. The salt retards the flame, allowing the candle wax to be consumed by the flame before the wick is consumed. This ensures a steady supply of wax to the flame.

Wicks for Candlemaking

There are three kinds of braided wick available for beeswax candlemaking: cored wicks, flat wicks, and square wicks.

Cored wicks are braided around a central stiff core that keeps the wick upright when surrounded by a pool of wax. They are usually used for jar candles, votive candles, and tea light candles that are meant to be fully consumed by the flame. The central core may be made of wire, stiff paper, or cotton. The wicks have a round profile.

They are often sold cut to length, with a wick tab already attached to the base of the wick, making them easy to insert into containers. If you purchase these in a skein of wick, you will need to cut them to length and insert them into wick tabs before using them.

Bloom on Beeswax

All 100 percent beeswax candles will develop a whitish bloom over time. The bloom is a sign of the quality of the beeswax. This is caused by natural oil in the wax that rises to the surface. Warmth causes the oil to blend with the wax once again. On smooth candles, simply brush the surface of the candle with a soft cloth. The friction of the cloth will warm the wax and cause the bloom to dissolve back into the wax. On candles with an intricate surface design, pass a warm hair dryer briefly over the surface to restore the original color. Or, you can leave the bloom as a testimony that the candles are 100 percent pure beeswax.

Flat wicks are braided using three bundles of fibers. They are the most commonly used wicks for taper and pillar paraffin candles sold to the consumer. Flat wicks are not commonly used in beeswax candles due to their tendency to clog and extinguish the flame.

Rounder and sturdier than flat wicks, **square wicks** are the best wick for beeswax pillar and taper candles. They don't clog as easily when used with beeswax, fragrance, and dye additives.

Braided wicks have a top and a bottom. To find the top of the wick, examine the braid closely. On one side of the braid, you'll see interlocking Vs in a column along the length of the wick. Hold the wick so that the V is right side up, and your wick will be right side up. An upright, braided wick naturally bends over into the flame, becoming self-trimming in the combustion zone of the flame. A downside wick splays in the flame, forming a bead of carbon on the top of the wick. This is called "mushrooming." It may not self-trim in the flame.

Wicks used with votive candles, jar candles, and tea lights often have a metal core so that they will stand upright in the holder. These wicks burn hotter than uncored wicks, allowing the wax to be completely consumed. The metal core used to be made with lead wire, but zinc is more commonly used today. Lead wicks give off lead fumes when they combust. Metal core wicks may not self-trim, as the metal core prevents the wick from curling over on itself.

HOW TO DETERMINE WICK SIZE TO USE WITH CLEANED YELLOW BEESWAX

Candle Size	Wick Size	Weight of Beeswax per Candle	Approximate Burn Time	Amount of Essential Oil per Candle (for Scent)
Tea light	2/0	0.5 ounce	4 hours	12 drops
Votive	3/0	2 or 3 ounces	15 to 23 hours	50 drops
¾ to ⅞-inch-diameter taper	#2	2 ounces	10 hours	50 drops
1.5 to 2-inch-diameter pillar	#2	3 ounces (varies by height)	7 hours x height in inches	0.5 teaspoon
2 to 2.5-inch-diameter pillar	#3	8 ounces (varies by height)	12 hours x height in inches	1.5 teaspoons
2.5 to 2.8-inch-diameter pillar	#4	9 ounces (varies by height)	16 hours x height in inches	2 teaspoons
2.9 to 3.2-inch-diameter pillar	#6	12 ounces (varies by height)	25 hours x height in inches	2.5 teaspoons
3.3 to 3.5-inch-diameter pillar	#7	16 ounces (varies by height)	33 hours x height in inches	1 tablespoon

Wick Size

The size of wick used when making candles is important. Candle wicking comes in various sizes to accommodate small tea lights to 3-inch-diameter pillar candles. When the candle wick is the correct size for the diameter of the candle, the candle is dripless and smokeless. When a candle wick is too small for the candle, the candle will drip because the wick cannot burn the wax as fast as it is pooling. When a candle wick is too large, the wick will smoke because the flame consumes the wax faster than the wax can melt. If the flame flickers on the candle, your candle wick is too large for the diameter of the candle. It can't get enough fuel to feed the flame. You'll need to remake the candle with a bigger wick.

Candle wicks are sized according to the number of strands of cotton thread in each wick. A 2/0 wick is smaller than a #2 wick. Candle wicks *increase* in size from #0 to #7, but *decrease* in size from #0 to 2/0, 3/0 etc. The wicks with the "/0" are more tightly braided. The wicks with the "#" in front are more loosely braided, which allows the diameter of the wick to increase without increasing the weight of the wick.

Those who live at elevations higher than 2,000 feet may need larger wicks in their candles. Since the air is thinner at higher elevations, there is less oxygen to burn in the candle flame. Consider using a wick one or two sizes larger if you live at higher elevations.

Making Candles with Beeswax Sheets

Making candles from beeswax sheets is an easy introduction to candlemaking. The soft, honey smell of the beeswax is intoxicating as you work with it. The colors are pleasing. A wide variety of candle sizes and shapes can be made using just beeswax sheets.

Some books and websites suggest that you add scent to rolled beeswax candles by soaking the wick in essential oils. This isn't a good idea for a couple reasons. First, essential oils are flammable and could cause the wick to burn faster than the wax, extinguishing the flame. Also, the oils can interfere with the wick's uptake of the wax, causing your candle to sputter and burn out prematurely. The honey scent of beeswax sheets doesn't need additional scent.

Beeswax sheets are sold as comb foundation for beekeepers. While beekeepers are limited to a variety of undyed sheets for their comb foundation, these sheets also come in dozens of bold and pastel-dyed colors. Expect to pay around $2 per 8½ x 16-inch sheet from most bee suppliers, with the price going down for bulk purchases of 50 sheets or more. One beeswax sheet will make a pair of 8-inch taper candles.

Rolled Taper Candles

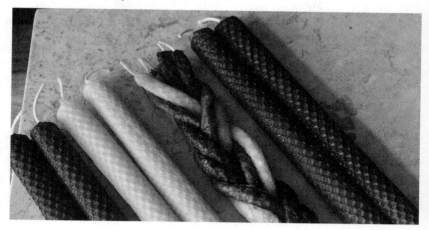

These are the first beeswax candles many people learn to make. They are perfect for making in a group setting. I've made them with groups of individuals as young as 6 years of age. Kids should work on this project with adult supervision.

YIELD: 1 pair of 8-inch taper candles per sheet

MATERIALS

1 beeswax sheet in color of choice

2 (9-inch) #2 wicks

EQUIPMENT

Scissors or craft knife

Ruler

Hair dryer

DIRECTIONS

Note that the beeswax sheet has a grain. As you are working with the beeswax sheet, you'll want to make sure that both your candles have the same grain pattern and are oriented in the same direction.

1. Use the scissors to cut the beeswax sheet in half on the long edge to make two rectangles that are 8½ x 8 inches. Your wicks will line up along the 8-inch side of this rectangle.

2. Work with one half-sheet of wax at a time. Using a hair dryer, gently heat the wax only until it becomes soft and pliable. Don't heat it so long that it begins to melt.

3. Find the upside of the wick. Lay the wick along the 8-inch edge of one beeswax sheet, lining up the bottom end of the wick with the end of the piece of wax. The top of the wick will overhang your beeswax sheet.

4. Using your fingers or the edge of a ruler, firmly fold the edge of the wax candle over the wick. Begin to roll the wick up into the candle, making the roll as tight as possible around the wick to exclude air. Use caution as you roll so that you don't crush the hexagonal cells on the outside of the wax.

5. When you get to the end of the wax, apply more heat from the hair dryer to soften the unrolled edge. Press the edge of the wax to seal it against the body of the candle. Roll the candle against a hard surface to seal and correct the shape of the candle. One candle is finished.

6. Repeat steps 3 to 5 with the other half of the beeswax sheet, ensuring that the wick is upright in the candle and the bottom of the wick is even with the bottom of the wax sheet along the 8-inch side of the wax.

7. Allow the candles to sit for 48 hours before burning.

🐝 Rolled Birthday Candles

Do you cringe when you see the neon wax droplets pooling on chocolate icing? Why settle for dyed paraffin candles for your family birthday cakes when you can make nontoxic, sweet-smelling, beeswax birthday candles like these?

YIELD: 48 (2⅛-inch) birthday candles

MATERIALS

1 beeswax sheet

3 yards 5/0 wick

EQUIPMENT

Ruler

Craft knife

Cutting mat

Hair dryer

DIRECTIONS

1. Laying the beeswax sheet on a cutting mat, score a line every 2⅛ inches along the short side of the beeswax sheet, using your ruler and craft knife. Use the marks to divide the sheet into four equal 2⅛ x 16-inch pieces.

2. Working with one beeswax strip at a time, measure in 1¼-inch intervals, marking them along the 16-inch length of the strip. Cut each strip into 12 sections that are 1¼ x 2⅛ inches. You now have 48 rectangles.

3. Cut the wick into 48 2½-inch-long pieces. Since birthday candles burn only briefly, it's not necessary to establish the direction of the wick.

4. Begin with the first piece of wax, positioning it so that the longer side extends from left to right on the table. Soften the wax with a hair dryer until it is just barely glistening. Line up the bottom of the first wick with the left side of the wax, along the long edge, closest to you. The top of the wick will overhang the right side of the wax by three-eighths of an inch. Using the edge of a ruler, turn up the long side of the softened wax closest to you at a right angle to the table.

5. Begin to roll the candle with your thumb and forefinger, away from yourself. Roll the candle as tightly as you can so that there are no air pockets around the wick. Keep the bottom of the candle even. When you get to the end, use the warmth of your hands to seal the edge of the candle.

6. Repeat steps 4 to 5 with the other 47 rectangles and wicks. It takes longer to read these directions than it takes to actually make the candles, so don't be intimidated. Your family deserves beeswax candles on their birthday cakes.

Rolled Chanukah Candles

Chanukah candles are used in the *chanukiah*, the special nine-candle menorah that is lit on each of the eight nights of Chanukah. The candles are left to burn until they burn out on their own. The candles are required to be large enough to burn for a minimum of 30 minutes on weeknights and a minimum of two hours on Friday night. Each night, fresh candles are placed in the chanukiah. On the first night of Chanukah, a single candle is lit, along with a helper candle called the "shamash." The shamash is replaced each night with a fresh candle and is used to light the other candles. On the second night of Chanukah, two candles are lit with the shamash. One extra candle is lit each night until the chanukiah is fully lit on the eighth night of Chanukah.

You'll need 44 candles to complete the festive ceremony for the 8 days. Chanukkiot vary in the size of candles needed. Most use small candles that are much smaller than tapers, but larger than birthday candles. You may need to measure your own chanukiah to determine how big to make your Chanukah candles. These measurements are based on the two chanukkiot I have.

These beeswax candles are 4 inches long and burn for 1½ to 2 hours—long enough to eat dinner and play some games.

YIELD: 44 (4-inch) Chanukah candles

MATERIALS

3 beeswax sheets, honeycombed or patterned in the colors that you like

5½ yards 2/0 wick

EQUIPMENT

Cutting mat

Ruler

Craft knife or sharp scissors

Hair dryer

DIRECTIONS

1. Lay your first beeswax sheet on the cutting mat. Using your ruler and craft knife, score a line every 4 inches along the long side of your beeswax sheet. Use these marks to divide the sheet into four equal 4 x 8½-inch pieces. Repeat with the remaining two sheets. You will end up with 12 rectangles. (Note: Reserve one of the 4 x 8½-inch rectangles. You won't need it for this project.)

2. Working with your first strip, measure in 2⅛-inch intervals along the 8½-inch length of the strip. Cut the strip into four sections that are 2⅛ x 4 inches. Repeat with the remaining 10 strips for a total of 16 pieces from each beeswax sheet (except on the last sheet, as noted above), or 44 total.

3. Cut the wick into 44 4½-inch lengths.

4. Position the first piece of wax so that the longer side extends from left to right on the table. Soften the wax with a hair dryer until it is just barely glistening. Line up the bottom of the first wick with the left side of the wax, along the long edge closest to you. The top of the wick will overhang the right side of the wax by half an inch. Using the edge of a ruler, turn up the long side of the softened wax closet to you at a right angle to the table.

5. Begin to roll the candle with your thumb and forefinger, away from yourself. Roll the candle as tightly as you can so that there are no air pockets around the wick. Keep the bottom of the

candle even. When you get to the end, use the warmth of your hands to seal the edge of the candle. Roll the candle on the table to correct any unevenness.

6. Repeat steps 4 and 5 with the other 43 rectangles and wicks.

7. Follow your family traditions in using and lighting these Chanukah candles for a meaningful family celebration.

🪰 Havdalah Candles

Havdalah candles are intricate candles that make lovely hostess gifts and wedding gifts for Jewish or Messianic Christian families. The Havdalah candle is the candle that is used during the ceremony that marks the end of the Shabbat rest and the beginning of a new week in a Jewish or Messianic home. It is a braided candle with a minimum of three wicks and often as many as six or more. It is important that the wicks are close enough together that when lit, the flame from each wick merges into one fire that resembles a torch.

For this project, you'll roll six thin candles to make each Havdalah candle. Then you'll link them together, while still warm, into a flat braid. The base of the candle can be molded to fit into the candlestick that you have, or you can use a special candlestick intended to hold the rectangular shape of the Havdalah candle.

YIELD: 4 Havdalah candles

MATERIALS
3 beeswax sheets in three different colors
6 yards 2/0 wick or 1½ yards per candle

EQUIPMENT
Ruler
Craft knife or sharp scissors
Hair dryer

DIRECTIONS

1. Using your ruler and craft knife, divide each beeswax sheet into eight 2 x 8½-inch rectangles. You'll have 24 rectangles with eight of each of three colors.

2. Cut 24 wicks 9 inches long. Determine the top of the wicks by looking for the V pattern in the wick.

3. Make your first candle. Pick two rectangles of each color and set the rest aside. Lay out one of the rectangles with the long side extending left to right on the table. Place the bottom of one wick flush with the left edge of the rectangle in front of you. This will be the bottom of the candle. Lay the length of the wick along the 8½-inch side of the wax. About one-half inch of wick will overhang the top end of the candle.

4. Using a hair dryer, lightly warm the wax, just until it glistens. Using a ruler, push up the wax until the long edge closest to you is perpendicular to the table surface and begins to curl over the wick.

5. Using your fingers, roll the wax tightly around the wick. Use the warmth of your hands to seal the open edge of the candle against the candle body. Repeat with the other five rectangles.

To braid the Havdalah candle

1. Take all six thin candles and line them up, keeping their tops even. Press them tightly together side by side. It's alright to curve them in slightly, so that when they are lit the flames join into one more easily.

2. Working with two strands at a time, begin to braid the candles from the top toward the center, beginning at the wick end of the candles, just as if you were braiding a child's hair. I found it easier to work with one candle strand and then bring the partner candle strand along following it.

3. You may need to soften the candles again with the hair dryer to keep them pliable. When you get to 3 inches from the bottom of

the candle, begin to work with each strand separately, continuing to braid in a pleasing pattern. As you get close to the bottom of the candle, stop braiding and even up the bottom of the candle, using the warmth of your hands to curve the candle into a tight round or rectangular end that will fit your chosen candle holder.

4. Repeat steps 2 to 8 to make three more candles from the remaining 23 wicks and 18 wax rectangles.

5. It does take some practice to get a beautiful Havdalah candle, but it's worth it, and you can burn the practice pieces so none of your practice is wasted. Once you have this technique mastered your friends will be begging you to make them these sweet and beautiful candles.

🌿 Christmas Tree Candles or Ornaments

These small, conical candles resemble a fir tree. Use them for gift toppers, tree ornaments, party favors, or table settings for your winter holiday decorations.

YIELD: 4 (4-inch) Christmas tree–shaped candles

MATERIALS

1 dark green beeswax sheet

½ yard plus 8 inches 1/0 wick

EQUIPMENT

Ruler

Craft knife or sharp scissors

Hair dryer

DIRECTIONS

1. Lay out the beeswax sheet so that the long side extends from left to right on the table. Measure 4¼ inches along the 8½-inch side of the beeswax sheet. Score the sheet at this point, dividing the sheet in half. Use the craft knife or scissors to cut the sheet

in half. You'll have 2 pieces of beeswax measuring 4¼ inch x 16 inches.

2. Working with half of the beeswax sheet at a time, place the rectangle on the table in front of you with the long side extending from left to right on the table. Using the craft knife, score a diagonal line from half an inch up from the bottom of the rectangle, beginning at the left side, to half an inch down from the top of the rectangle on the right side. Separate at the score mark. Repeat with the other rectangle. You now have four right-angle triangles that are 3⅝ inches on the shortest side.

3. Find the top of your wick by looking for the V along the braid. Cut the wick into 5-inch pieces if you are making candles to burn. If you are making ornaments for gift toppers or to hang on a Christmas tree, make the wicks 6 inches long.

4. Lay your first triangle on the table in front of you with the point of the triangle pointing away from you and the 3⅝-inch edge closest to you. Place the right angle of the triangle on your left side. Place the wick along the short edge of the triangle with the bottom of the wick flush with the right-angle corner. The top of the wick will overhang the wax sheet by 1 or 2 inches.

5. Warm the wax with the hair dryer until it just begins to glisten. Do not overheat. Using the edge of a ruler, turn up the short edge of the wax and fold it over the wick. If you are making an ornament or gift topper, you'll need a loop in the top of the tree rather than a wick. To make the loop, take the candle wick and fold it over, capturing the end in the tree top on the next roll of the candle wax and leaving a small loop hanging out the top. Be sure the end is securely captured in the wax. Roll the candle tightly, keeping the bottom even and letting the sides of the candle flare out slightly. Secure the edge by warming the wax with your hand and pressing firmly.

6. Repeat with the three remaining Christmas tree shapes.

TIP: Add glitter to decorate the tree shapes. To do so, warm the trees with a hair dryer. Sprinkle a small amount of glitter on a paper towel (use polyester glitter rather than aluminum glitter if the candles will be lit). Roll the warmed wax in the glitter to evenly distribute on the wax. Shake off excess glitter. Allow the trees to harden.

🐝 Cookie Cutter Ornaments

When my daughter was three years old, we made these ornaments for Grandma. Since Grandma was on oxygen, she no longer used candles, but she cherished these handmade ornaments until she passed away, keeping them beside her wedding china and her mother's silver teaspoons in her china cabinet.

These are easy enough for a child to make. Preschool children may need a little help getting the edges even.

YIELD: 1 ornament or candle per beeswax sheet

MATERIALS

Beeswax sheets in various colors

7 inches 1/0 wick for each ornament or 4 inches of 1/0 wick for each candle

EQUIPMENT

Cutting mat

Cookie cutters in seasonal holiday shapes, like stars, angels, Santas, gingerbread men, hearts, bunnies, chicks, etc.

Hair dryer

DIRECTIONS

1. Lay out the first beeswax sheet in front of you on the cutting mat. Using the cookie cutter shape of your choice, press down on the beeswax. Repeat on the same sheet of beeswax until you have eight cutouts for each ornament. If you are making several ornaments of the same style, you can stack the sheets and cut through all of them at once, being careful to impress the shape through all layers.

2. Warm one cutout with the hair dryer, then place another cutout of the same shape on top. Press together. Warm the wax and press a third layer on top of the first two. Warm the third layer and press a fourth layer on top of this.

3. To make an ornament, take the wick and double it over, laying the end in the middle of the ornament and leaving the loop out of the top by at least half an inch. To make a candle, place the wick snugly in the middle of the wax shape, leaving ½ inch of wick out of the top. Place a fifth layer over the wick to secure it. Correct the alignment of the cookie cutter shapes if necessary to make a neat package.

4. Warm the ornament again and press the final layers in place, warming it between each layer to get a good wax seal.

5. Hang the ornament using the loop at the top or tie the ornament to a gift by slipping a ribbon through the loop. If you are making a candle, secure it in an appropriate candle holder before lighting.

6. Repeat steps one to four to make ornaments or candles using additional beeswax sheets and cookie cutters.

Hand-Dipped Candles

Hand-dipped candles are the height of the chandler's art. A perfectly formed taper has smooth sides and a uniform shape. It speaks of handmade artisan craft. Hand-dipped tapers are lovely to burn and a treasure to gift. They can be made in any size, from small birthday candles to long 16-inch, wedding tapers. Your only limitation is the size of your dipping pot.

Hand-dipped tapers require cleaned yellow beeswax that is without impurities but retains a honey scent and a fine yellow color. Filtered and bleached white beeswax is often used for wedding candles.

Lower quality beeswax should not be used for hand–dipped tapers. The impurities will clog the wick and mar the uniform shape of the candle.

When dipping candles, it's a good idea to have a second container of melted wax, of the same quality, to top up the dipping pot as it empties so the candles don't get too cold during the layering process.

A pound of beeswax yields approximately 20 fluid ounces, or 2½ cups of melted wax.

🐝 Hand-Dipped Candles

All hand–dipped candles need the same equipment and use the same method, regardless of the size of the finished candle. Please don't put the wax in the microwave to melt it. You can't control the temperature of the wax that way. In addition, any impurities in the wax can cause it to overheat, breaking down the crystal structure and integrity of the wax and making it unsuitable for candles. Instead, use the double boiler method described here.

YIELD: Varies

MATERIALS

Cleaned yellow beeswax

Wicks in the appropriate sizes

EQUIPMENT

Drop sheet

Newspaper or other absorbent material

Deep wax pot

Stock pot

Candle drying rack—I use a wooden clothes drying rack with a drop sheet under it

Wax Cautions

Beeswax melts between 140°F and 147°F. Temperatures over 185°F discolor beeswax and damage the crystalline structure of the wax. The flash point of beeswax is 400°F. Never let your beeswax get that hot. The ideal dipping temperature for beeswax is 155°F to 165°F. If it's too hot, the wax will not congeal around the wick. If it's too cold, you'll get a pebbling texture on the sides of the candle instead of a smooth surface.

DIRECTIONS

1. Prepare your work space by laying down a drop sheet on the floor and covering your work area with newspaper or other absorbent layers. (If you do accidentally spill beeswax, d–limonene, a natural solvent derived from orange oil, will dissolve it and make cleanup easier. Test the surface, though, before using it, to ensure that the surface is safe to use with d–limonene.)

2. Create a double boiler using a deep wax pot. Fill the stock pot with water so that the water comes half way up the side of the wax pot. Place it on the stove top. Fill the wax melting pot with cleaned yellow beeswax.

3. Simmer on low to medium heat until the wax liquefies. This can take several hours. Be patient.

4. Cut your wick to appropriate lengths, 1½ to 2 inches longer than the candle you want to make. Check the direction of the wicks and place them so that the V is upright. If you are dipping pairs of tapers, tie two wicks that are oriented in their upright direction at the top, using a half hitch knot. Do not use one long wick and fold it in half. You will dip the two wicks together in the wax pot, making two candles simultaneously.

5. Hold the wicks at the knot. Prime the wicks by dipping them into the wax pot to saturate them with beeswax. Do this at least three times, allowing the wax to harden on the wick between dipping. Straighten the wick by holding the top of the wick in your fingers and pulling down on the bottom of the wick, firmly.

You won't need a weight to hold the wick straight in the pot, because the weight of the wax will hold the wick down once you dip it several times.

6. To make a pair of dipped candles, hold the wicks at the knot and lower the wicks quickly into the melted wax. Hold the wicks in the wax for 30 seconds. Remove them slowly from the dipping pot, holding the candles over the pot until the wax solidifies and they are no longer dripping. You should see a buildup of wax on the candle. If not, lower the temperature of the wax by 5°F. Between dips in the wax pot, hang your candles over the drying rack, till they harden. Each candle will require several dips in the wax to build up enough layers of wax to form the candle.

7. Periodically roll the solid but warm candle on a marble slab or other firm surface to straighten the candle and correct its shape before dipping again.

TROUBLESHOOTING

Problem	Possible Cause	Solution
Lumpy surface on the candle	Wax is too cold	Increase wax temperature by 5°F Re-dip before the candle has cooled fully
Wax is not building up	Wax is too hot	Decrease wax temperature by 5°F
Air pockets between layers	Wax is too cold	Increase wax temperature by 5°F Keep candle warmer between dips
Candle misshapen	Wick was not straightened between dips	Roll the candle on a firm surface while warm to straighten the taper

🐝 Dipped Taper Candles

Melt your wax as directed in Hand-Dipped Candles (page 36). Once your wax is melted, you're ready to make tapered candles.

YIELD: 10 pairs of 9-inch tapers

MATERIALS

5½ pounds beeswax

6 yards #2 wick

EQUIPMENT

Craft knife or sharp scissors

Candle drying rack—I use a wooden clothes drying rack with a drop sheet under it

Marble slab or other firm surface

DIRECTIONS

1. Dipped tapers require a wick that is 2 inches longer than your finished candle. To make a 9-inch taper, cut your wicks 11 inches long. Look for the upright V along the wicks and orient two wicks into their upright position. Tie a knot at the top, securing two wicks together.

2. As directed in Hand-Dipped Candles recipe on page 36, prime the 10 pairs of wicks using beeswax and set them aside to harden.

3. Dip the first pair of candles by placing them into the dipping pot quickly. Hold them in the dipping pot for 30 seconds. Remove them slowly from the dipping pot, holding the candles over the pot until the wax solidifies and they are no longer dripping. You should see a buildup of wax on the candle. If not, lower the temperature of the wax by 5°F.

4. Place the dipped candles on the drying rack. Allow to cool between dips. Some people recommend cooling the wax quickly by dipping into a pail of cold water. However, I don't recommend speeding up the cooling process. The water can be encapsulated in the wax and this will affect the wicking of the wax, possibly causing poor burning. Patience is a virtue in chandlery.

5. Repeat steps 3 to 4 for the remaining nine paired wicks, keeping the dipping pot topped with hot wax to within 1 inch at the top.

6. Periodically roll the solid but warm candle on a marble slab or other firm surface to straighten the candle and correct its shape before dipping again.

7. Continue dipping and cooling until your candles are about ⅞ inch in diameter or until they fit your chosen candlesticks.

🐝 Hand-Dipped Birthday Candles

Hand-dipped birthday candles are miniature versions of dipped taper candles.

YIELD: 48 birthday candles

MATERIALS
3 cups melted wax, divided
4 yards 1/0 wick

EQUIPMENT
Deep tin can
Craft knife or sharp scissors
Rod for cooling the candles
Marble slab or other firm surface

DIRECTIONS
1. Create a double boiler using a deep tin can (page 15). Melt the first 2 cups of wax in the can by simmering over medium heat until the wax melts. The wax should come to within 1 inch of the top of the can.

2. Each candle will be 2 inches long. Since birthday candles burn only briefly, it's not necessary to establish the direction of the wick. Use the craft knife to cut the wick into 24 5-inch lengths. Each wick will make 2 birthday candles approximately 2 inches long. The birthday candles are dipped in pairs. Fold the first wick in half and dip into the can to prime. Straighten each end of the wick, keeping the wick folded and the candles paired.

Allow it to cool. Dip the wick again. Straighten the ends of the wick after each dip, while keeping the wick folded. Repeat for the remaining 23 wicks.

3. Dip the first pair of wicks in the melted wax quickly, holding the wicks in the wax for 15 seconds and pulling them out slowly. Hang the pair of wicks over a rod to cool while you dip the other pairs of wicks.

4. Repeat the dipping process two more times until your candles are the approximately $3/16$ of an inch wide.. Each candle pair will be dipped five times. Straighten the candles by rolling them on a smooth surface, like a marble pastry board.

5. Add the extra wax to the can when the level of the wax in the can is below half and you are no longer able to dip the candles to their full heights. This will ensure that all the candles are the same length.

6. Allow to cool for 24 to 48 hours before using.

🦟 Shabbat Candles

Shabbat candles are the candles lit on Friday night in observant Jewish households. The candles should burn for at least 3 hours and no more than 5 hours, which should be enough time to burn out on its own. The candles are not extinguished. Dipped tapers are not suitable for Shabbat candles, since they have a longer burn time and would be a fire hazard if left burning unattended. Instead, shorter candles are used that are about 4 to 5 inches tall and no more than ¾ inch in diameter.

YIELD: 12 (4-inch) Shabbat candles with a 4-hour burn time

MATERIALS

2 yards 2/0 wick

12 ounces beeswax, plus 2 pounds to top off the melting pot

EQUIPMENT

Craft knife or sharp scissors

Marble slab or other firm surface

DIRECTIONS

1. Using the craft knife, cut 12 5½-inch-long pieces of wick. Find the direction of the wicks by looking for the upright V in the braid of the wick. Tie pairs of wick together at the top, with both wicks in their upright orientation. Follow the dipping instructions for Dipped Taper Candles (page 38), completing the dipping when the candles are three-quarters of an inch in diameter.

2. Correct the shape by rolling on a marble slab or other firm surface while still warm.

3. Allow the candles to set for 48 hours before using.

Twisted and Shaped Candles

With hand-dipped candles, one advantage over molded candles is the ability to manipulate the shape of the candle while it is still warm. Taper candles may be manipulated into fancy shapes like spirals or braids. These are especially meaningful for wedding candles, where two candles may be formed into one candle with two wicks joining into one flame. Try some of the following special effects.

🐝 Twisted Spiral Candles

These are made from two tapers that are no more than half an inch in diameter at the base and still warm from the dipping pot. The two tapers will be twisted around each other as the two wicks remain even at the top. The bases are pressed together and shaped into a ⅞-inch round to fit into a candle holder. The twisted tapers will then be dipped a final time to secure them and make them look more connected.

Three-, four-, and five-strand plaits and spirals may be made using this technique. Each strand in the multi-strand taper should be a quarter of an inch or smaller in diameter so that the base of the finished candle is no more than seven-eighths of an inch in diameter to fit in a standard candle holder.

🐝 Flattened Tapers

These candles look like twisted spirals, but instead of being made from two tapers, they are made from a single taper. Basically, a completed taper candle that is of the correct finished diameter is rolled flat with a rolling pin on a firm surface while it is still warm. The bottom end is left round so that it will fit in a candle holder. The top and the bottom of the flattened taper are twisted so that it forms a spiral. This overall shape may be straightened as necessary, then allowed to cool completely.

🐝 Luminaries

Luminaries are not actually candles, but rather, candle holders. Luminaries are meant to be placed outside in the darkness to light the way. Luminaries are often lit with tea lights. They should be translucent to allow light through.

While you're dipping tapers and have the wax melted in the dipping vat, make a few luminaries to place outside along your garden path.

Luminary wax doesn't need to be the same high-quality wax as tapers and candles; making them out of the leftover wax after candlemaking is a good use of otherwise wasted wax.

YIELD: 1 luminary

MATERIALS

1 water balloon filled with water

2 pounds melted beeswax

Dried flowers (optional)

EQUIPMENT

Parchment paper

12 x 17 inch baking sheet

Deep wax pot

DIRECTIONS

1. Place parchment paper over a baking sheet to hold your completed luminaries while they harden. Fill the water balloons with cold water and secure the top. The size of the balloon will be the size of the base of your luminary.

2. Create a double boiler using a deep wax pot, with an opening large enough to accept a filled water balloon. Warm the beeswax to 155°F. The luminary will take 2½ ounces of beeswax. The extra wax is to give enough depth to the dipping pot to make dipping easier.

3. Hold the water balloon by the tie and dip it to three-quarters of the way up the body of the balloon. Place on the parchment paper to flatten the bottom of the balloon and stabilize.

4. Dip the balloon, leaving it in the dipping vat for 30 seconds and then removing to allow excess wax to drip back into the vat. Flatten the bottom of the luminary by placing it firmly on the parchment paper so that it is stable and level. Continue to dip five to eight more times, flattening the bottom between dips. The shell of the luminary should be thin to allow light to pass through radiantly. The bottom should be thicker than the sides to offer stability and safety.

5. When the wax has hardened but before the wax has fully cooled, hold the balloon over the sink and cut the tie on the balloon to let the water out. Slip the balloon out of the luminary. Allow the luminary to cool completely.

6. To use the luminary, place a tea light in a plastic holder into the bottom of the luminary. (Tea lights with metal holders get hot enough to melt the bottom of the luminary.) Place the luminary

in a safe place on a stone or brick, where the heat from a candle will not cause a fire and where pets or children cannot disturb the burning candle. Ensure there are no dry grasses that could catch fire, as well.

7. Luminaries can be decorated on the outside with dried flowers or glitter. Press the dried flowers into the wax while it is still warm. Give it one final dip to coat the plant material and bond it on the outside of the luminary.

Molded Candles

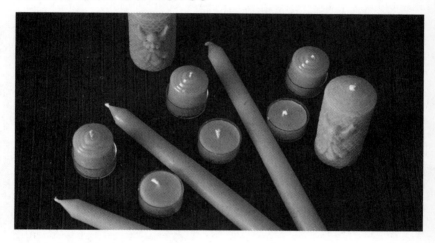

Molded candles offer an incredible variety of shapes and sizes to encourage your creativity and enhance your decor. From making simple tea lights to intricate figurines in wax, all you need is an appropriate mold to speed up the candlemaking process and make one-of-a-kind gifts for family and friends. You may even enjoy it so much you'll decide to start a home-based business.

My first candle mold was a reproduction of an antique tin mold for making taper candles. The mold had eight cavities and the candles were strung in pairs. There was no Internet in those days, but I had volume three of *The Family Creative Workshop*. In that encyclopedia of craft, there was a brief two-page article that explained how to use tin molds, with grainy black and white photos that were difficult to decipher. I didn't know anyone who made candles, but how hard could it be? Well, as it turns out, it wasn't easy.

Looking back now, it was amazing that my candles even burned cleanly. I didn't know about sizing the wick to the diameter of the candle (see the How to Determine Wick Size to Use with Cleaned Yellow Beeswax chart on page 23). I naively cut a length of wick double the size of the candles I wanted, plus a few inches to fit over the gap between two candle cavities in the mold, from a spool of wick I picked up at the local five-and-dime store. I knotted the end of the wick to plug the hole at the end of the cavity. Luckily I thought to lay down newspaper over the counter before I poured the hot, liquid wax. As fast as I poured the wax into the eight cavities, it came out the bottom of the mold and pooled on the newspaper.

In my second attempt at making molded tapers, I plugged the wick hole with candle putty and poured the wax. The wax didn't leak out. The mold was solid. I chilled the mold in the freezer to encourage the candles to contract in the mold. But the candles didn't pop out of the mold. I ended up banging the sides of the mold with a hammer to get the candles to drop out.

After that I tried greasing the mold with petrolatum, tallow, and olive oil. I finally found silicone mold release spray. Silicone candle molds are much easier to use than the antique tin molds, though silicone molds are more expensive to purchase.

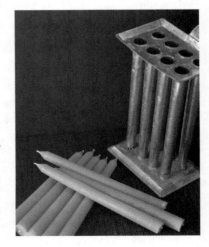

Mold Preparation

Whether you use tin molds, silicone molds, or rubber molds, preparing the mold is important to your success. Each mold is a little different, so learn the idiosyncrasies of your mold material. Tin and plastic molds that make candles need to be sprayed with mold release spray. Beeswax shrinks when it cools and pulls away from the sides of the mold. However, mold release spray ensures that the design is clean and the surface unblemished when the candle is unmolded. The wick is placed in the mold after the mold is sprayed. The silicone in the mold release spray can clog the wick and inhibit the fuel uptake from the wick during burning.

Antique Tin Molds

Antique tin molds are quite attractive decor pieces. They are often sold for decor and aren't used as much today for candlemaking, having been replaced by plastic and silicone molds. If you purchase one to use as a candle mold, buy it from a reputable chandler supply. Then you'll be sure that the seams on the mold are soldered for candlemaking and can take the heat of melted wax.

Taper Candles

Tin taper candle molds come with four, six, eight, or up to twelve cavities. Tin molds were used in colonial times to speed up the home manufacture of beeswax and tallow candles. Today these molds are being replaced by novelty silicone molds; however, new tin molds are still available at beekeeping and candle suppliers.

The cavities in the molds are paired and a single strand of wick is sometimes used to thread all the cavities. However, as we learned earlier in the chapter, the wick has a top and a bottom. Candles will burn better if the wick is in the correct orientation in every cavity. I recommend that you take the time to cut individual wicks, as done here.

Tin molds come in shiny tin and galvanized tin models. Choose shiny tin for beeswax candlemaking when possible. The galvanized surface causes beeswax candles to look dirty, as the zinc coating is lifted off by the mildly acidic nature of the beeswax.

Tapers, made in ½- and ⅞-inch sizes so that they fit in standard candle holders, have a long burn time of about an hour per inch of candle.

YIELD: 8 (10-inch, 2.5-ounce) candles

MATERIALS

3 yards 2/0 wick

3 cups beeswax

EQUIPMENT

10-inch taper candle mold with 8 cavities

Mold release spray

Craft knife or sharp scissors

Darning needle

Mold sealant putty

8 bobby pins

Deep wax pot

Spoon

DIRECTIONS

1. Before you thread the wick, spray each cavity in the mold with silicone mold release spray.

2. Using your craft scissors, cut eight pieces of wick 13½ inches long.

3. Determine the V along the first wick. Holding the top, dip the wick into the melted beeswax. Leave the top 3 inches of wick free of the wax. The beeswax coating will stiffen and prime the wick, making it easier to thread through the mold. Repeat with the other seven wicks.

4. Thread the top of one wick through the darning needle. Drop the threaded needle into the mold cavity, point-side down. The needle will fall through the wick hole in the bottom of the candle mold. Pull the wick through the hole, just to the point

where the wax begins on the wick. Leave the waxed part of the wick inside the mold. Note that the bottom of the candle mold cavity is the top of the candle.

5. Secure the top of the wick in the hole of the mold using an overhand knot. Secure the bottom of the wick in the center of the mold using a bobby pin. Repeat with the remaining seven wicks, dropping one into each of the remaining seven cavities.

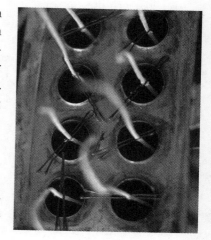

6. Using mold sealant putty, seal the wick hole at the bottom of each cavity on the outside of the mold, enclosing the wick at the point that it exits the hole. Do this for each wick. Your candles are now ready to be poured.

7. Create a double boiler using a deep wax pot with a spout. Melt 3 ounces of beeswax per cavity. Fill the mold with the wax, taking care to keep the wicks centered. Tap the side of the mold with a spoon to encourage any bubbles to rise to the surface. Set the mold aside while it cools. Do not speed up the cooling time. After 10 minutes, check the area around the wicks. If the wax is dimpled, add fresh wax to the mold around the wicks. Wait 10 minutes and add more wax to fill the depression if the candle around the wick dimples.

8. The wax will shrink as it cools. When the sides of the tin mold are no longer warm to the touch, place the mold in the freezer briefly. This will encourage the candles in the mold to contract, making it easier to remove them from the mold. Remove the sealant putty from over the knots at the base of the mold. Untie the knots in the wicks before you remove the candles from the mold.

9. Polish the tapers with a soft cloth to remove any imperfections. Sometimes the seam from the tin mold will be visible on the candle. The friction from polishing may remove this. Trim the wicks from the bottom of the candles. True the candle bottoms by rubbing them against a hot surface, like a flat frying pan or pot, lined with parchment paper, to ensure that the bottoms are even and the candle will stand level. One 10-inch beeswax taper will burn for approximately 10 hours.

✳ Votive Candles

Votive candles are intended to be fully consumed by the flame. Always burn votive candles in a flame-safe container that is large enough to hold all the melted wax.

Tin votive candle molds require a special wicking technique. They do not have a wicking hole and look like tin cups. A wick pin is used in each tin votive cup. The wick pin is placed in the mold before the candle is poured to hold the place for the wick in the wax as the wax cools. The wick pin is removed after the candle cools. A special cored wick with a wick tab is inserted in the candle, into the hole left by the wick pin.

YIELD: 6 (3-ounce) votive candles

MATERIALS

2½ cups beeswax

6 prepared wicks with tabs

EQUIPMENT

6-cavity votive mold or 6 tin votive mold cups

6 wick pins

Mold release spray

Deep wax pot with spout

Candles and the Church

Beeswax candles have been used in Christian worship since at least the fourth century, both for light and as a symbol in worship. While tapers, pillar candles, and votive candles have a place in liturgy, votive candles are the only kind lit by the people (see Types of Candles on page 20). Votives are symbolic of the sacrifice of prayer. In some traditions, the candle must be lit for the prayer to be heard by God, with the behavior of the flame acting as an indication that the prayer was accepted.

From earliest times, beeswax candles were limited in use to the rich and the clergy; the poor would use less expensive tallow candles in their homes. Because tallow was smoky and burned poorly, the church mandated beeswax candles for religious purposes. Votive candles had to be purchased from the clergy. In some parishes, families kept beehives in their gardens to meet the household need for both honey and beeswax. These families paid their tithes and taxes to the church in wax. In other parishes, monasteries controlled the production of both beeswax and candlemaking. Even today there are monasteries making beeswax candles, using the wax donated by church members.

DIRECTIONS

1. Spray the candle mold and the wick pins with mold release spray. Place one wick pin in each mold. This will center the wick placement in each votive candle.

2. Create a double boiler using a deep wax pot with a spout. Melt the beeswax over medium heat.

3. Pour beeswax into the votive mold or tin cups. Set the molds aside to cool. As the wax cools, it will shrink around the wick pin. Add more wax to fill the space. Once the wax in the molds are fully solid and cold to the touch, unmold the votive candles.

4. Remove the wick pin by turning the candle upside down and pressing on the point of the pin. The wick pin will slide out of the candle, leaving a centered hole for the wick to be threaded into.

5. Prepared wicks have a stiff center core and a wick tab. Push the wick from the bottom of the votive candle to the top, through the hole left by the wick pin when it was removed from the candle. Trim the wick so half an inch remains on top. Polish the candle with a soft cloth. Candles should be set aside for 48 hours before burning to allow the crystal structure of the wax to harden.

Plastic and Glass Molds

Plastic and glass molds are meant to be used as candle molds as well as candle holders. The burning candles form a pool of melted wax as the candle burns. The container holds the melted wax and prevents spills while ensuring safe burning.

🐝 Tea Lights

Tea light candles are a must for ambient lighting during holidays and special evenings at home. Each one has its own cup made of plastic or metal, so that the wax can melt completely. Tea lights get their name because they were originally used under a teapot to keep it warm. They are also

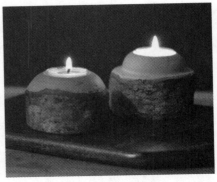

used as food warmers, for fondue, and for warming scented oil. Tea light holders can be made of glass, metal, or wood, because the tea light stays relatively cool while the candle burns. Tea lights made with metal holders can get hot enough to burn skin, since the heat of the melted wax is conducted by the metal. Plastic tea light holders remain cooler to the touch, even with melted wax in the cup.

Each tea light holds half an ounce of beeswax and burns for four to five hours. When burning tea lights, leave the candle burning for at least two hours to establish a pool of wax before extinguishing.

If the wick is blown out too soon, the candle will not consume all the wax on future burns.

Tea light wicks are best with a zinc core. Zinc core wicks are stiff and stand upright in the wax cup without support. Further, zinc wicks burn a little hotter, allowing all the wax to melt in the cup and ensuring a complete burn, with no residual wax wasted.

YIELD: 27 to 30 tea lights

MATERIALS

2 cups beeswax

1 tablespoon essential oils (optional)

30 metal wick tabs

4 feet 2/0 zinc core wick

30 tea light cups

EQUIPMENT

Glass measuring cup

Craft knife or sharp scissors

12 x 17-inch baking sheet

Parchment paper

DIRECTIONS

1. Create a double boiler using a glass measuring cup. Melt beeswax in the glass cup over medium heat. Add 1 tablespoon of essential oils per 2 cups of melted beeswax when making tea lights, if desired. While the beeswax is melting, prepare the wick tabs with the wick.

2. When threading the wick through the wick tab, check the direction of the wick. The wick should be upright in the tab to ensure that it bends into the flame and self-trims for a clean burn. You can save time by threading all the tabs onto the wick at once.

   To thread a wick through a metal wick tab, dip the end of the wick in melted wax. Use your fingers to pinch and smooth the wax on the wick to stiffen it, like the end of a shoelace. The wick will now be firm enough to push through the hole in the tab without the aid of a hook or a needle. Thread all the tabs on the wick prior to cutting the wick into individual lengths.

3. Using a craft knife, cut each wick to 1½ inches, including its pre-threaded tab. Fold one-quarter to one-half inch of the bottom of the wick under the tab. Dip the bottom of the tab in melted beeswax. Press the tab firmly into the bottom of the tea light cup, centering it, being sure to trap the bottom of the wick under the tab. Repeat with each wick. Each tea light cup has a circular embossing on the bottom of the cup to help center the wick tab. The melted wax will hold the wick tab in place long enough for you to pour the hot wax into the tea light cup. Prepare as many tea light cups in this manner as you plan to fill. Two cups of melted wax will fill 27 to 30 tea lights.

4. Prepare a baking sheet by lining it with parchment paper to catch any drips. Cold wax will peel off the parchment paper easily and can be re-melted. Place the empty, prepared tea light molds on the lined baking sheet. Straighten the wicks inside the tea light cups before filling.

5. Fill each cup with melted wax to just below the brim. If you are using plastic tea light cups, you'll be able to hold each tea light in your hand as you fill it. If you are using metal tea light cups, the metal transfers the heat of the melted wax to the cup. You will need to leave metal tea light cups on a heat-protected surface to fill them. Fill slowly to avoid spills. As the wax cools, it may contract around the wick. Allow the candle to solidify. But while it is still warm, top it up with fresh wax to fill in the depression around the wick. Cool completely.

6. If the wax in the tea light cups cools too quickly, it may crack around the wick as it's cooling. Pour more melted wax over the top of the candle to seal any cracks.

Freshly poured candles are still molten, even when they appear to be solid. It takes a few days for them to recrystallize into solid wax. Tea lights will burn best after they have cooled for at least 24 hours, giving the crystal structure time to reestablish in the wax.

🐝 Mason Jar Candles

A Mason jar candle is easy to make and adds a beautiful glow to the ambiance of a winter evening. Mason jar candles use a prepared wick, with a wick tab to set the wick into the bottom of the jar.

YIELD: 1 (8-ounce) candle

MATERIALS

7 ounces beeswax

6 inches #4 wick

1 wick tab

1 (8-ounce) decorative mason jar

1½ teaspoons essential oil (optional)

EQUIPMENT

Glass measuring cup

2 chopsticks

Skewer (optional)

DIRECTIONS

1. Create a double boiler using a glass measuring cup. Melt the beeswax in the glass cup over medium heat. While the beeswax is melting, prepare the wick tab with the wick facing up. Dip the bottom end of the wick into the melting beeswax. Pinch the end between your thumb and finger to create a firm end, like the end of a shoelace. Slide the end through the wick tab from the top. Secure the wick tab in the center of the bottom of the jar using a small amount of melted beeswax.

2. Center the wick in the jar using two chopsticks across the top of the jar to hold the wick steady.

3. When the beeswax is melted, add the essential oil to the melted wax, if using. Pour the beeswax into the jar, slowly. Center the wick after pouring, if necessary. Reserve 2 ounces of wax to add after the wax in the jar has firmed up.

4. After 10 minutes, when the beeswax has formed a crust on the top of the candle, use a chopstick or skewer to pierce the wax around the wick. Top up the candle with more beeswax to fill in any air holes around the wick. Repeat this again in 10 or 15 minutes.

5. The candle should cool for a full 24 to 48 hours to allow the crystal structure of the wax to reform. This candle will burn for about 36 hours.

🐝 Candle in Silicone Mold

Silicone molds come in a wide variety of shapes and sizes. Some of them are strictly novelty figures and are not meant to be burned. Others are very detailed pillar candles that are a pleasure to give and receive as gifts. For candles intended to be burned, look for shapes that are even all around the candle, such as beehives, decorated pillars, and decorated tapers. Avoid odd shapes or asymmetrical designs. These won't burn evenly.

Silicone molds are flexible and do not need to be sprayed with mold release. The molds can be used over and over again. The results are beautiful and detailed. However, the molds can be a significant investment.

YIELD: 1 candle

MATERIALS
#2 wick that is 2 inches longer than candle mold

Beeswax

EQUIPMENT
Silicone mold

Flat elastic bands

2 chopsticks

DIRECTIONS

1. Measure the wick according to the height of the mold. Determine the upright V on the wick and note the top of the wick. The top of your candle will be at the bottom of the silicone mold. Slip the top of the wick into the bottom of the mold, at the base of the slit that opens the mold. Allow a half inch to remain outside of the mold.

2. Secure the mold closed by slipping elastic bands around the mold at half-inch intervals, ensuring that the seam in the mold is closed along its full length.

3. Secure the wick in the center of the top of the mold using two parallel chopsticks.

4. Melt enough beeswax to fill the mold, plus an extra quarter cup. The beeswax will shrink as it cools. Fill the mold with melted beeswax. Adjust the wick if necessary to keep it centered in the candle. After 10 minutes, the wax around the wick will dimple. Add more wax to fill in any hollows or dimples that appear as the wax cools.

5. Allow the candle in the mold to cool completely before removing the candle from the mold. Silicone molds usually have intricate details, which need time to solidify. Smaller candles are usually ready to remove from the mold within 60 to 90 minutes.

Make Your Own Silicone Mold

Making your own silicone molds is an affordable way to obtain a variety of candle shapes without investing a lot of money. When you make your own molds, you can customize the shape of your candles. The mold material is a two-part epoxy designed specifically for mold making. I used an antique apothecary bottle for my custom silicone candle mold.

YIELD: 1 or 2 molds

MATERIALS

Hot glue

Mold release spray

Silicone 2-part epoxy mold medium

EQUIPMENT

24-ounce plastic vessel

Object to mold, such as a decorative glass bottle

12-inch wooden paint stick

Craft knife

DIRECTIONS

1. Size the vessel to hold the mold medium according to the size of your object to be duplicated so that you don't waste mold material. Ideally, you want about 1½ inches of silicone all the way around your mold material and over the top of your mold. This will give you a stable mold that is resilient and durable. You'll need a vessel like a 24-ounce yogurt container to hold the object being duplicated. Anchor your object being duplicated with a spot of hot glue in the center of the bottom of the vessel. Spray the mold shape and the holding container with silicone mold release spray.

2. Mix the two-part silicone mold material according to the manufacturer's directions, using a wooden paint stick. Pour over the object in the vessel, being sure to cover the top of the object with at least 1½ inches of silicone. If the object you are duplicating is an open vessel, cover the opening with a lid to prevent the molding compound from entering the vessel. This will become the top of your candle. Gently tap the container on a hard surface to remove any air bubbles. Allow the mold to

set for the length of time recommended in the directions on your specific molding product.

3. Remove the silicone material from the molding vessel. Using a sharp craft knife, slice a clean line through only one side of the silicone material to release the object being duplicated. Once the object is removed, cut a clean line to the center of the bottom of the mold (the top of your candle), through the silicone, to create an anchor in the center for the wick.

4. Clean up the bottom of the mold so that it will be fit for pouring wax into. Your mold is ready for use.

Once the two-part silicone molding material is mixed it must be used immediately. Have enough vessels with models ready so that none of it is wasted. The unmixed silicone mold material has a shelf life. Only buy the amount that you can use up within six months.

Use your custom mold as you would any silicone candle mold. Completed molds last indefinitely.

Chapter 3

BEESWAX FOR PERSONAL CARE

Pleasant words are like a honeycomb, sweet
to the soul and medicine to the bones.

—Hebrew proverb

Thirty to 40 percent of the world's trade in beeswax is used in cosmetics and personal care. However, beeswax makes up only about 4 percent of worldwide wax products because most commercial cosmetics use other waxes, like paraffin and carnauba wax, in their manufacture.

Why beeswax and beauty? Because beeswax is moisturizing and skin conditioning. In skin-care products, it holds therapeutic elements in suspension. Beeswax also mediates the texture and malleability of skin care and cosmetics. It is emulsifying, allowing for the blending of oil- and water-based ingredients. It solidifies liquid oils at room temperature, making them easier to use and to store. These benefits have been recognized throughout history.

Beeswax, almond oil, and roses were some of Cleopatra's cosmetic ingredients. She bathed in milk and rose petals. Then she slathered on scented lotion and cream to preserve her acclaimed beauty, with beeswax as a central ingredient. Beeswax was also used in Egypt as a hairstyling agent, much as we use pomade today.

In the second century, the Greek doctor Galen offered his patients "cold cream" made with beeswax, water, and olive oil, scented with roses. Roman women used the doctor's cold cream for their complexions, and the practice of improving complexions with herbs, olive oil, and beeswax was passed on through the generations, little changed until the modern manufacturing era.

For hundreds of years, households from cottage to castle contained a "still-room" off the kitchen, where the woman of the house created herbal cosmetics, medicines, cleaning products, fermented drinks, perfumes, food preserves, and liqueurs from her garden bounty. Wealthy homes had large rooms set aside to make and store the finished products, while smaller homes had a large closet off the kitchen. Women kept handwritten stillroom recipe books containing their best recipes, passed down from mother to daughter.

While today most people go to the drugstore, grocery store, or big-box store to buy the cosmetics that they need, in times past it was a normal household task to make these necessities at home. The cosmetics and personal care recipes in this chapter will show you how to once again make these products yourself.

Sometimes we think of cosmetics as products that beautify, like lipstick, bronzer, and blush, while personal care items are the products that make us acceptable in society, like toothpaste, soap, and deodorant. But in reality, every product that enhances our health and improves our well-being is contributing to that inner glow that shines through the eyes and enhances our beauty. For the sake of organization, I've divided the recipes into natural cosmetics (lip balms, lipsticks, and balms/moisturizers) and personal care products (perfumes, deodorants, nail care, massage products, and emulsions/lotions). First, let's cover some information you'll find useful when making these recipes.

Seasonal Formulations

Beeswax gives hardness to personal care products. The hardness or tackiness can be manipulated by changing the percentage of beeswax in the recipe. Why is this important? You may want to change the formulation of a lip balm, making a harder lip balm that resists melting in the summer and a softer lip balm that melts easier in the winter. When you make your own personal care products, you can control the softness or hardness, the slip, and the stickiness of the finished product.

The beeswax isn't the only variable in the final consistency of the product, though. Vegetable fats like cocoa butter, shea butter, or mango butter offer some firmness to the final product, whereas the liquid oils can provide slip, richness, or a speedier absorption rate.

Herb-Infused Oils

One advantage of making your own cosmetics and personal care products is the ability to customize each recipe to meet your own needs. The recipes I've created here use liquid oils that are infused with medicinal herbs like calendula, elderflower, dandelion blossoms, rose petals, and other herbal allies. These herbs help your skin heal itself. They soften, encourage cell proliferation, and reduce itching or dryness. The herbs, combined with oils, butters, and beeswax, help your body to balance itself.

How to Make an Herb-Infused Oil

Most of these recipes begin with herb–infused oils. There are two ways to make herb–infused oils:

The slow way to infuse oil. The easiest way is to fill a jar halfway with dried herbal material, such as lavender blossoms. Pour olive oil or sweet almond oil over the top of the plant material. Place the jar on a blender base and whirl to chop up the dried plant material, making a slurry. Remove the blender base and recap with the jar lid. Set the jar aside for two to four weeks in a warm place, shaking daily or as often as you think of it.

After the infusion period is up, strain the plant material out of the oil using a cheesecloth. Squeeze the cheesecloth to recover as much of the oil as possible. The oil closest to the herb is richest in the herbal components that you want in the oil. Reserve the oil. The plant material can be composted.

The fast way to infuse oil. You can also infuse oil with herbs using heat. While this method is faster, there are less active compounds in the finished oil than there are when using the slow method. Nevertheless, sometimes you need infused oil immediately and you don't have time to wait a month.

Create a double boiler using a glass measuring cup. Place the required amount of herbs in the measuring cup. Add the required amount of oil. (Unless otherwise stated, 2 tablespoons of dried herb mixed with 4 tablespoons of oil will be sufficient for the recipes that follow.) Cover the measuring cup with plastic wrap to retain any volatile oils in the plant material. Simmer, covered, over low heat for one hour. Turn off the heat and allow the oil to come to room temperature naturally.

Strain the plant material out of the oil using a cheesecloth or a fine strainer. Press the plant material to recover as much of the oil as possible. Retain the oil. Compost the herbs.

Prepping Herbs for an Oil Infusion

Ideally, most plant material used to make infused oil will be completely dry. Introducing moisture from fresh plants into the oil can cause the oil to spoil or go rancid. St. John's wort is the exception to this rule. It should be macerated in oil while fresh, but the blossoms should be wilted for a day before being added to the oil, to reduce the chance of mold. St. John's wort oil is a deep garnet red color when properly made.

If you need infused oil quickly and you don't have time to wait for the plant to dry before proceeding, here's a shortcut. When using fresh plant material to make infused oil, allow the herbs to wilt for several hours or overnight before proceeding. Use the fast method for infusing the oil with the herbs when using fresh plant material, in most cases. The additional heat will allow some of the water in the plant material to evaporate out of the oil, reducing the chances of rancidity. Note that the finished oil won't be as strong as when using the long method with dried herbs.

Adding Cosmetic Colors to Beeswax

Beeswax can be easily blended with oils but not with water. So any colors that you add to beeswax need to be able to be used in oil-based products. Adding water-soluble colors, like beet root powder, to beeswax and oil mixtures will result in disappointment.

Colors that are insoluble will be dispersed in your finished product but won't dissolve in your medium, whether it is oil based, water based, or emulsified. The colors will remain suspended in the solution.

Working with powdered colorants can be messy. Colors can become airborne. Work in a well-ventilated space. Wear a dust mask or ventilator and gloves. Clothing and work surfaces should be protected from staining.

There are five classes of colorants for use in cosmetics:

Botanicals. These colorants are extracted from plants. Some are water soluble, like beet root powder, and some are oil soluble, like paprika. The catalog description for each botanical colorant will state whether it is soluble in oil or water. Oil-soluble botanicals are best to use with beeswax.

Botanicals have a tendency to fade with time and with exposure to light. Their color can shift with changes in pH. Because they are a natural product, the color may be different between batches. The color can vary between suppliers as well. Rose hip extract is a botanical colorant.

Clays. Because clays are naturally occurring mineral deposits, their color can vary from batch to batch. They are insoluble in both oil and water. Clays are available in earthy shades of green, pink, brown, red, beige, and white. The color remains true over time. Only a small amount is needed to give color to a cosmetic.

Clays are best when mixed with oils in cosmetic preparations. When they are mixed with water, they have a tendency to draw moisture from the skin. They flake as they dry if mixed with water, much like a facial mask.

Use clays as no more than 5 percent of the cosmetic batch. Use 1 tablespoon per pound in cold processed soap.

Oxides. Oxides occur naturally as oxidized metals like iron rust and ocher. However, because of the risk of heavy metal contamination in naturally occurring oxides, the oxides sold for mineral makeup and as a soap colorant are synthesized colors that are chemically identical to the natural product. They are insoluble, reliable, light, reproducible, and inexpensive.

They are stable in a wide range of pH concentrations and do not fade over time, making them ideal for use in cosmetics. Oxides are potent colors. A little goes a long way. Begin with $1/32$ of a teaspoon in cosmetic formulations and increase the amount until the desired color is achieved. In cold-processed soap, use one-quarter to one-half teaspoon per pound of finished soap.

Ultramarines. Ultramarines are similar to oxides in every respect except that they do not occur in nature. They are synthetic pigments. You may find them useful to bring a touch of coolness to a blend. Ultramarines offer blue, purple, plum, and lavender shades that aren't available in other colors. Ultramarines, like oxides, are potent colors, so use sparingly.

Micas. Insoluble in both oil and water, micas add a shimmery touch to cosmetics. They are available in every hue, but their color comes from FD&C dyes, so they aren't a natural product. If you want to limit your cosmetics to natural colors you can purchase silver or pearl mica and tint them with oxides to get the color you want. Use micas as .01 to 1 percent of the cosmetic batch.

Mix the colors separately in a resealable bag. Make adjustments to the color by adding ¹⁄₆₄ of a teaspoon of additional oxide colors. Make notes so that you can repeat the colors that you prefer. Then, when the color pleases you, add the color packet to the cosmetic base. Oxide and mica colors can also be added to nail polish base to get matching makeup.

The Best Double Boiler for Making Cosmetics

When melting beeswax for small batches of cosmetics, create a double boiler using a glass measuring cup. Glass is the least reactive of the options for melting beeswax. Refer to page 14 for instructions on creating a double boiler.

Cleanliness

When making natural cosmetics, you have the best chance of minimizing microbial contamination by starting out clean. Start with clean hands and clean utensils. Wipe your work surface with antimicrobial cleaner. Sanitize your bowls and utensils. Should any of your handmade cosmetics smell "off," develop mold, or show other signs of spoilage, toss them out and make a new batch.

Generally, cosmetics made with an oil base and no added water have a long shelf life of a year or more at room temperature. If you find signs of contamination in oil-based cosmetics, examine your procedures. Cosmetics like lotions that include a water fraction have a limited shelf life and should be kept refrigerated. Make these in small batches. Expect to remake water-based lotions on a monthly basis.

Those who make cosmetics for sale will need to comply with their country's cosmetic manufacturing regulations, which may necessitate making products in a commercial kitchen as well as follow mandated procedural record keeping.

Natural Cosmetics

Natural cosmetics preserve moisture, protect our skin, and provide a barrier against external pollution and toxins. As you go through the recipes in this section, you'll see a pattern:

Beeswax + vegetable butter + herb-infused oil + specialty additions = product

The recipes vary in their proportions of these ingredients and in their consistency. Harder products contain more beeswax and butters; softer products contain more liquid oils. The specialty ingredients add scent, luxury feel, slip, nutrients, or color.

Lip conditioners like lip balm and lipstick are moisture barriers that seal in the precious moisture in your lips, soothe chapped lips, and protect from moisture loss in the elements. Sometimes a simple lip balm is all that's needed, but in harsh weather conditions extra moisture, as well as protection from the weather, may be what you're looking for.

✳ Cool Mint Lip Balm

This refreshing peppermint lip balm tastes good while providing moisturizing protection for your lips. It glides on smoothly with the addition of silk protein and rich mango butter. Rose

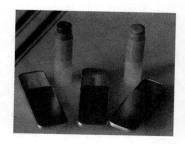

hip oil offers antioxidant defense to soothe and protect your vulnerable lips.

YIELD: 4 to 5 lip balm tubes or 2 (½-ounce) tins

INGREDIENTS

2 teaspoons beeswax

1 teaspoon mango butter

2 teaspoons calendula-infused olive oil

½ teaspoon rose hip seed oil

Pinch silk protein powder

10 drops peppermint essential oil

DIRECTIONS

1. Infuse calendula flowers in olive oil using one of the methods mentioned in How to Make an Herb-Infused Oil (page 62).

2. Make a double boiler using a glass measuring cup. Gently simmer the beeswax, mango butter, and calendula-infused olive oil in the cup until the beeswax and mango butter are liquid. Stir to blend well. Remove from the heat.

3. Allow this mixture to cool until it is just warm to the touch. Stir while it is cooling to prevent it from setting too quickly. Stir in the rose hip seed oil, silk protein powder, and peppermint essential oil. Stir well to incorporate.

4. Pour into lip balm tubes or lip balm tins. Allow the mixture to cool completely before using. Label and date.

🐝 Fairy Glitter Lip Balm

Little princesses love fairy glitter to apply to their arms, cheeks, and lips. This is completely nontoxic and won't make them sick if they lick it. The ingredients are simple and inexpensive so you can make a double batch for birthday party favors, gifts for all the cousins, or even granddaughter gifts. Mix a batch up in just 15 minutes.

If you choose to use it, the natural rose hip extract gives this lip balm a pretty pink color in the container. But on the skin, the pink is barely noticeable. This is perfect for the little princess that loves to be pretty, without the high color of grown-up makeup.

YIELD: 3 to 4 lip balm tubes

INGREDIENTS

1 teaspoon beeswax

1 teaspoon cocoa butter

1 teaspoon coconut oil

¼ teaspoon rose hip extract (optional)

¼ teaspoon silver mica

Pinch titanium dioxide

10 drops sweet orange essential oil

DIRECTIONS

1. Make a double boiler using a glass measuring cup. Gently simmer the beeswax, cocoa butter, and coconut oil in the cup until the beeswax and cocoa butter are liquid. Stir to blend well. Remove from the heat.

2. Allow this mixture to cool until it is just warm to the touch. Stir while it is cooling to prevent it from setting too quickly. Stir in rose hip extract (if using), mica, titanium dioxide, and sweet orange essential oil. Stir well to incorporate.

3. Pour into lip balm tubes or lip balm tins. Allow the mixture to cool completely before using. Label and date.

🐝 Lip Balm Sunscreen (SPF 15)

You need more than a moisturizer in your lip balm if you are working outside in the summer heat or playing hard at the beach or on the slopes. Commercial sunscreen contains toxic and carcinogenic ingredients, like retinyl palmitate, a synthetic form of vitamin A that actually encourages malignant cells to develop; PABAs;

and oxybenzone, a hormone-disrupting chemical that is absorbed through the skin. When you put it on your lips, you're likely to swallow it, too. No, thank you.

This natural sunscreen lip balm contains raspberry seed oil for an SPF of 15. SPF, or sun protection factor, is a measure of how well a sunscreen blocks UVB radiation, but says nothing about UVA radiation. UVA is the kind of radiation that goes deep into your tissue. To increase the protective barrier to SPF 20, add zinc oxide, which protects against both UVA and UVB radiation.

YIELD: 4 to 5 lip balm tubes or 2 (½-ounce) tins

INGREDIENTS

1 teaspoon calendula-infused olive oil

2 teaspoon beeswax

1 teaspoon refined shea butter

½ teaspoon rose hip seed oil

1 teaspoon raspberry seed oil

¼ teaspoon vitamin E oil

10 drops peppermint essential oil

½ teaspoon zinc oxide powder (optional)

DIRECTIONS

1. Infuse calendula flowers in olive oil using one of the methods mentioned in How to Make an Herb-Infused Oil (page 62). Make a double boiler using a glass measuring cup. Melt the beeswax and shea butter in the measuring cup. Stir to combine. Add the calendula-infused oil. Continue to heat and stir until the beeswax mixture combines with the oil. Remove from the heat.

2. Allow this mixture to cool while stirring with a spatula to prevent it from setting. Stir in the rose hip seed oil, raspberry seed oil, vitamin E oil, and essential oil. Stir to combine.

3. If using, stir zinc oxide powder into the oils with a spoon. Once the zinc oxide powder is moistened, use a whisk to combine fully. Please, use a dust mask and gloves when handling zinc oxide to protect against inhalation. Once it is incorporated into your lip balm ingredients, there is no safety hazard.

4. Spoon this into lip balm tubes or tins. Allow to set fully before using. Label and date.

✳ Chocolate Winter Sports Lip Balm

On the slopes, playing hard, you need more protection than the average lip balm can provide. This winter sports lip balm has shielding power and a bit of color. Plus, it tastes like chocolate. What's not to like?

Without the addition of zinc oxide, this sunscreen recipe has a natural SPF of about 15 and offers protection from UVB radiation only. To create a broad spectrum sunscreen and increase the SPF to 20, add zinc oxide to the recipe after the oils are mixed.

YIELD: 4 to 5 lip balm tubes or 2 (½-ounce) tins

INGREDIENTS

1 teaspoon chamomile-infused oil

2 teaspoons beeswax

1 teaspoon cocoa butter

½ teaspoon dark chocolate

½ teaspoon sea buckthorn seed oil

½ teaspoon rose hip seed oil

1 teaspoon raspberry seed oil

¼ teaspoon vitamin E oil

10 drops vanilla absolute (optional)

¾ teaspoon zinc oxide powder (optional)

DIRECTIONS

1. Infuse chamomile flowers in sunflower or olive oil using one of the methods described in How to Make an Herb-Infused Oil (page 62).

2. Make a double boiler using a glass measuring cup. Simmer the beeswax, cocoa butter, and dark chocolate in the measuring cup until the beeswax and cocoa butter melt. Stir to combine. Add chamomile-infused sunflower oil to the cup. Continue to heat and stir until the beeswax mixture combines with the oil. Remove from the heat.

3. Allow the mixture to cool while stirring with a spatula to prevent it from setting. Stir in the sea buckthorn seed oil, rose hip seed oil, raspberry seed oil, vitamin E, and vanilla absolute, if using. Stir to combine.

4. If using, stir zinc oxide powder into the oils with a spoon. Once the zinc oxide powder is moistened, use a whisk to combine fully. Please, use a dust mask and gloves when handling zinc oxide to protect against inhalation. Once it is incorporated into your lip balm ingredients, there is no safety hazard.

5. Spoon this into lip balm tubes or tins. Allow to set fully before using. Label and date.

Rose Pink Lip Gloss

This lip gloss has a gentle sheen of pink on the lips, with the herbal moisturizing and astringent effect of roses. You'll want to infuse olive oil with fresh or dried rose petals to capture the fragrance of the blossoms in season. Then you'll be able to make this lip balm all year round.

Castor oil gives this lip gloss shine. The color comes from alkanet, a natural red color that is oil soluble. While it will give a translucent pink sheen to the lips, it is not a prevailing color.

YIELD: 3 (½-ounce) tins

INGREDIENTS

¼ cup castor oil

1 teaspoon alkanet root

2 teaspoons beeswax

2 teaspoons cocoa butter

1 tablespoon rose petal–infused olive oil

¼ teaspoon vitamin E oil

10 drops rose essential oil or 4 drops rose geranium essential oil

DIRECTIONS

1. Make castor oil infused with alkanet root by preparing a double boiler using a glass measuring cup. Place the castor oil in the measuring cup. Place the alkanet root in a heat-sealable tea bag. Place the bag in the oil. As the castor oil heats, it will draw the color from the alkanet root. Gently heat till the castor oil is the color that you want. When the recipe is complete, the lip gloss color will be lighter than it appears in the castor oil, so prepare a darker shade than you actually want in the finished lip gloss. Strain and reserve the dyed oil in a glass jar with a tight-fitting lid.

2. Place 1 tablespoon of the castor oil infused with alkanet root in a double boiler with a clean glass measuring cup.

3. Add beeswax and cocoa butter. Heat gently until the beeswax is melted. Stir the mixture together to blend well. Remove from heat.

4. Allow to cool, stirring so that the mixture doesn't set firmly. Once it is just warm to the touch, use a flexible spatula to stir in the rose-infused oil, vitamin E, and essential oil. Continue stirring until it is fully blended and the mixture has cooled to room temperature.

5. Spoon the lip gloss into tins. Label and date.

✴ Lip Balm with Shimmer and Shine

Sometimes you want a little glitter in your cosmetics. Mica reflects light and adds the shimmer that you crave. To any of the above lip balms or lip glosses, add one-eighth of a teaspoon of silver mica powder, or try this basic lip balm recipe.

YIELD: 4 lip balm tubes or 2 (½-ounce) tins

INGREDIENTS

2 teaspoons beeswax

1 teaspoon cocoa butter

1½ teaspoons olive oil

½ teaspoon castor oil

10 drops distilled lime essential oil

¼ teaspoon silver mica powder

DIRECTIONS

1. Make a double boiler using a glass measuring cup. Simmer the beeswax, cocoa butter, olive oil, and castor oil in the measuring cup on low until the beeswax and cocoa butter are melted. Stir to combine. Turn off the heat.

2. Continue to stir while the mixture cools naturally. Add essential oil. When the mixture is just warm to the touch and beginning to solidify, stir in the mica powder. Beat with a whisk to fully integrate the mica powder with the beeswax mixture.

3. Spoon into lip balm tubes or tins. Allow to solidify before using. Label and date.

✴ Basic Lipstick Base

This Basic Lipstick Base is used in the next three recipes. It's technically a lip balm, but the addition of titanium dioxide changes lip balm into lipstick, making the colors more opaque. Lip balm colors are usually transparent but when titanium dioxide is mixed in, the colors seem to darken. You don't need much to have a profound effect on the color. Magnesium stearate, which you will see in the following recipes, helps your lipstick stay on your lips. The butters and oils in this base can be changed according to your preference, provided the proportions remain the same. See Chapter 10 (page 258) for substitutions.

INGREDIENTS

2 teaspoons beeswax

1 teaspoon cocoa butter

1 teaspoon mango butter

1 teaspoon castor oil

1 teaspoon avocado butter

DIRECTIONS

1. Create a double boiler using a glass measuring cup. Melt the beeswax, cocoa butter, mango butter, castor oil, and avocado butter together in the double boiler.

2. Use immediately with the color base of your choice.

🐝 Winter Plum Lipstick

This lipstick is a rose leaning toward the purple shades. Play with the mineral colors inside a resealable plastic bag to find the shade you like best. Take good notes so that you can repeat the color at will.

YIELD: 4 to 5 lip balm tubes

INGREDIENTS

1 recipe Basic Lipstick Base (page 74)

Color Base

$\frac{1}{32}$ teaspoon titanium dioxide

⅛ teaspoon magnesium stearate

¼ teaspoon silk protein

⅛ teaspoon red oxide pigment

Pinch blue oxide pigment

10 drops spearmint essential oil

DIRECTIONS

1. In a resealable bag, place the titanium dioxide, magnesium stearate, silk protein, and red and blue pigments. Zip the bag and gently massage it with your fingers to full blend it. Stir the blended powders into your oil and beeswax base. Blend thoroughly.

2. Add essential oil. Mix well.

3. Pour into lip balm tubes. Label and date.

🌿 Rose Red Lipstick

This uses the same lipstick base as the Winter Plum Lipstick, but with a change in color packet.

YIELD: 4 to 5 lip balm tubes

INGREDIENTS

1 recipe Basic Lipstick Base (page 74)

Color Base

$\frac{1}{32}$ teaspoon titanium dioxide

$\frac{1}{8}$ teaspoon magnesium stearate

$\frac{1}{4}$ teaspoon silk protein

$\frac{1}{4}$ teaspoon red oxide pigment

1 teaspoon Australian red clay

10 drops peppermint essential oil

DIRECTIONS

1. In a resealable plastic bag, place the titanium dioxide, magnesium stearate, silk protein, red pigment, and clay. Zip the bag and gently massage it with your fingers to fully blend it. Stir the blended powders into your Basic Lipstick Base. Blend thoroughly.

2. Add essential oil. Mix well.

3. Pour into lip balm tubes. Label and date.

🐝 Cinnabar Lipstick

This uses the same lipstick base as the Winter Plum Lipstick, but with a change in color packet. This one leans toward the earthy tones.

YIELD: 4 to 5 lip balm tubes

INGREDIENTS

1 recipe Basic Lipstick Base (page 74)

Color Base

¼ teaspoon titanium dioxide

⅛ teaspoon magnesium stearate

¼ teaspoon silk protein

¹/₁₆ teaspoon yellow oxide

¹/₁₆ teaspoon brown oxide

1 teaspoon bronze mica

10 drops peppermint essential oil

DIRECTIONS

1. In a resealable plastic bag, place the titanium oxide, magnesium stearate, silk protein, oxides, and mica. Zip the bag and gently massage it with your fingers to fully blend it. Stir the blended powders into your Basic Lipstick Base. Blend thoroughly.

2. Add essential oil. Mix well.

3. Pour into lip balm tubes. Label and date.

Balms and oil-based moisturizers are mixtures of oils and waxes. No germicide is needed when making balms because there is no water added to the mixture. The liquid oils used in balms can be infused with herbs for their soothing, emollient, and demulcent actions. Even the weeds in your garden can be used to encourage skin repair and stop irritation or soreness. Each of the following recipes uses herb-infused oil for specific remedial actions. Use one of the methods for making herb-infused oil on page 62.

❀ Mineral Make-Up Bronzer

DIY bronzer contains none of the fillers and questionable cosmetic ingredients found in commercial products. It moisturizes as well as gives your complexion a healthy glow.

YIELD: 1 (1-ounce) container

INGREDIENTS

2 teaspoons beeswax

2 teaspoons mango butter

1 teaspoon jojoba oil

2 teaspoons rose hip seed oil

Color Base

½ teaspoon titanium dioxide

⅛ teaspoon magnesium stearate

¼ teaspoon silk protein

¼ teaspoon bronze mica

$1/_{32}$ teaspoon brown oxide

$1/_{64}$ teaspoon red oxide

$1/_{64}$ teaspoon yellow oxide

DIRECTIONS

1. Create a double boiler using a glass measuring cup. Melt the beeswax, mango butter, and jojoba oil together over low heat. Remove from the heat.

2. Using a whisk, stir in rose hip seed oil.

3. In a resealable plastic bag, place the titanium oxide, magnesium stearate, silk protein, mica, and the oxide colors. Zip the bag and gently massage it with your fingers to fully blend it. Adjust the colors if necessary to get the color that suits your own skin type. Stir the blended powders into your oil and beeswax base. Blend thoroughly. Mix well.

4. Pour into a 1-ounce push-up container. Label and date.

🐝 Calendula Hand Balm

Hand balm is a general moisturizer. It will feel greasy when first applied but will quickly absorb into the skin.

YIELD: 1 (4-ounce) jar

INGREDIENTS

2 tablespoons beeswax

2 tablespoons cocoa butter

3 tablespoons comfrey-infused olive oil

3 tablespoons calendula-infused olive oil

20 drops lavender essential oil

15 drops tea tree essential oil

DIRECTIONS

1. Create a double boiler using a glass measuring cup. Gently simmer the beeswax, cocoa butter, and infused oils in the cup until the beeswax and cocoa butter is fully melted. Stir to combine. Remove the measuring cup from the heat.

2. Allow the oil to cool slightly, stirring with a spatula to prevent the mixture from setting completely.

3. When mixture is just warm to the touch, add the essential oils. Stir to incorporate.

4. Pour into a 4-ounce glass jar. Cap tightly. Label and date.

🦟 Peppermint Foot Care Lotion Bars

These are solid lotion bars that are molded in the mold of your choice. I like to use a mold that allows the finished bar to fit into a recycled candy tin. These are easy to carry with you in a gym bag. They are a firmer bar that will stay solid at room temperature in most climates, yet they melt slightly when held in the hand.

These lotion bars are soothing and speed the restoration of cracked, rough heels and feet. Peppermint essential oil makes them stimulating; rosemary is antifungal and anti-inflammatory.

YIELD: 1½ cups or 6 lotion bars

INGREDIENTS

½ cup beeswax

½ cup shea butter

½ cup calendula-infused oil

¼ teaspoon peppermint essential oil

¼ teaspoon tea tree essential oil

¼ teaspoon rosemary essential oil

DIRECTIONS

1. Create a double boiler using a glass measuring cup. Simmer the beeswax, shea butter, and oils in the measuring cup just until the beeswax melts. Stir this together to incorporate the wax and the oils. Remove from the heat.

2. Stir while the mixture cools somewhat. When it is just warm to the touch and the mixture just begins to thicken, stir in the essential oils. Pour the mixture into six one-quarter cup silicone molds.

3. Allow the molds to harden at room temperature. Remove the bars from the molds. Wrap the bars in parchment paper and place in a tin. Label and date the tin.

TO USE

Hold the bar in warm hands until it just begins to soften. Rub the bar into your hands and then apply the amount that remains on your hands into your feet, being careful to apply to the heels and the balls of your feet.

🐝 Rose Facial Moisturizer for Older Skin

This is my favorite nighttime moisturizer. Roses are astringent and tighten older skin while softening and smoothing. This facial moisturizer uses cosmetic oils that are hydrating but are absorbed quickly into the skin, so they don't leave it feeling slick.

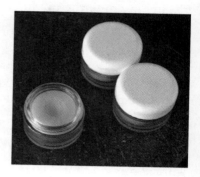

YIELD: 1 (4-ounce) jar

INGREDIENTS

1 tablespoon beeswax

2 tablespoons mango butter

2 tablespoons rose-infused olive oil

1 tablespoon rose wax

2 tablespoons pomegranate oil

1½ tablespoons rose hip seed oil

¼ teaspoon vitamin E oil

5 drops rose absolute or rose geranium essential oil

5 drops marjoram essential oil

DIRECTIONS

1. Create a double boiler using a glass measuring cup. Simmer the beeswax, mango butter, and rose-infused oil in the cup just until the beeswax melts. Stir this mixture together to incorporate the wax and the oils. Remove from the heat.

2. Add the rose wax and continue stirring until the rose wax is fully incorporated.

3. Stir in the pomegranate oil, rose hip seed oil, and vitamin E. Stir while the mixture cools somewhat.

4. When it is just warm to the touch and the mixture just begins to thicken, stir in the rose absolute and the essential oil. Keep stirring until the mixture is the consistency of pudding. Spoon this into a 4-ounce glass jar. Cap tightly, label, and date.

TO USE

Use as you would any facial moisturizer. It will feel slick when it is first applied but it will be quickly absorbed by your skin.

🜲 Body Butter for Everyday

This all-around moisturizer can be used on the face, hands, elbows, feet—anywhere you need a little extra buttering up.

YIELD: 1 (4-ounce) jar

INGREDIENTS

2 tablespoon beeswax

2 tablespoons shea butter

4 tablespoons calendula-infused sweet almond oil or olive oil

¼ teaspoon vitamin E oil

25 drops marjoram essential oil

15 drops lavender essential oil

DIRECTIONS

1. Create a double boiler using a glass measuring cup. Simmer the beeswax, shea butter, and calendula-infused oil in the cup just until the beeswax melts. Stir this together to incorporate the wax and the oils. Remove from the heat.

2. Stir in the vitamin E oil. Continue stirring while the mixture cools somewhat. When it is warm to the touch and the mixture just begins to thicken, stir in the essential oils.

3. Spoon the moisturizer into a 4-ounce glass jar with a tight-fitting lid. Label and date.

✳ Moisturizer for Oily Skin

Oily skin with acne can be painful. You don't need a heavy moisturizer. Rather, you need to find a balancing moisturizer that will allow the skin to breathe. These ingredients won't plug pores and the essential oils are antimicrobial, bringing your skin into balance.

YIELD: 1 (4-ounce) jar

INGREDIENTS

1 tablespoon beeswax

2 tablespoons mango butter

2 tablespoons mint-infused jojoba oil

1 tablespoon hemp seed oil

½ teaspoon sunflower lecithin

8 drops tea tree essential oil

10 drops rosemary essential oil

1 tablespoon aloe vera gel

DIRECTIONS

1. Create a double boiler using a glass measuring cup. Simmer the beeswax, mango butter, jojoba oil, hemp seed oil, and lecithin in the measuring cup on low heat until the wax is melted.

2. Remove from the heat and let cool until it is just warm to the touch. Add the essential oils. Using a hand held mixer or immersion blender, begin blending the beeswax mixture on low. Slowly drizzle the aloe gel into the beeswax mixture. Beat with the immersion blender for five minutes or until the mixture is uniform, thick, and creamy.

3. Spoon into a 4-ounce glass jar, label, and date. Keep refrigerated when not in use. This should be used within three to four weeks. Since there is no germicide in it, it will not keep at room temperature for more than two weeks without spoilage.

Personal Care

Personal care products allow us to be accepted in social situations, helping us to smell better, improving hygiene, and helping us shine. Personal care products are more intimate than cosmetics, often contacting our most sensitive skin. Ingredients used in personal care products should be nontoxic, organic, and of high quality. Personal care products directly affect our health and well-being.

Beeswax supports the structure of the other ingredients in each recipe, allowing personal care products like deodorants to slip into a tube, which can be twisted up for use, keeping the applicator clean. Beeswax preserves the scent of solid perfumes and improves the texture of moisturizers and creams.

🦟 Basic Solid Perfume

You can make a triple batch of this base using 2 tablespoons of beeswax and 6 tablespoons of jojoba oil, and then divide it to create three different perfumes by changing the essential oils that you use, or you may substitute one of the teaspoons of beeswax for a floral wax, like jasmine, rose, or mimosa to give a light base fragrance.

Consider packaging solid perfume in specialty lockets and small containers to showcase their specialness. A tiny but beautiful package has a greater perceived value when given as a gift.

YIELD: 1 (½-ounce) container

INGREDIENTS

2 teaspoons beeswax

2 tablespoons jojoba oil

80 to 100 drops essential oil

DIRECTIONS

1. Create a double boiler using a glass measuring cup. Simmer the beeswax and jojoba oil in the measuring cup over medium heat just until the beeswax is melted. Remove from the heat.

2. Allow this to cool to room temperature, stirring while it cools. When it is the consistency of soft butter, add essential oils a few drops at a time until the fragrance is pleasing.

3. Pour into a ½-ounce tin or desired container(s). Label and date.

TO USE

Apply to pulse points.

Notes on Making Your Own Perfume

Perfume and cologne are two of the more toxic personal care products on the market. Synthetic fragrance has been linked to dermatitis, asthma, insulin resistance, and even cancer. Perfumes and fragrances represent more than 3,000 undisclosed chemical compounds. Manufacturers are not required to list the actual chemicals on the label. Using these recipes, those with sensitivities to fragrance can create their own unique solid perfume blends based on scents that they tolerate well.

Beeswax helps keep volatile scents in suspension so they don't dissipate into the air as quickly. Perfumes are made up of a combination of lighter top notes, middle notes, and bass notes. The lighter top notes are generally the first thing you smell in a fragrance blend. Top notes also dissipate quickly. The middle note in a scent is the lingering note, and the bass note is the drone that can last for hours. Think of florals as providing the top notes. The middle notes are a combination of floral, grassy, and woodsy scents, with the bass notes coming from the wood and resin family of fragrances or strong florals like jasmine.

✤ Woodsy Perfume

With citrus top notes and deep wood and resin fragrance, this perfume has the exotic scent of sandalwood with lingering hints of smoke.

YIELD: 1 (½-ounce) tin

INGREDIENTS

2 teaspoons beeswax

2 tablespoons jojoba oil

25 drops sandalwood essential oil

25 drops grapefruit essential oil

30 drops bergamot essential oil

2 drops vetiver essential oil

10 drops cinnamon essential oil

DIRECTIONS

1. Create a double boiler using a glass measuring cup. Simmer the beeswax and jojoba oil in the cup over medium heat just until the beeswax is melted. Remove from the heat.

2. Allow this to cool to room temperature, stirring while it cools. When it is the consistency of soft butter, add the essential oils a few drops at a time until the fragrance is pleasing.

3. Pour into a ½-ounce tin. Label and date.

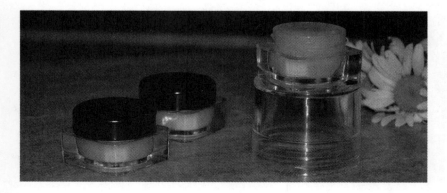

Apply to pulse points.

🦟 Floral Perfume

This recipe uses rose floral wax to replace half of the beeswax in the other solid perfume recipes. Floral wax is a by-product of absolutes produced from fresh blossoms. Floral waxes are soft vegetable waxes that retain the fragrance of the flowers they are extracted from. They are less expensive than floral absolutes and more within reach of most budgets.

YIELD: 1 (½-ounce) tin

INGREDIENTS

1 teaspoon beeswax

2 teaspoons jojoba oil

1 teaspoon rose wax

20 drops rose geranium essential oil

15 drops sweet marjoram essential oil

10 drop sandalwood essential oil

10 drops sweet orange essential oil

DIRECTIONS

1. Create a double boiler using a glass measuring cup. Simmer the beeswax and jojoba oil in the measuring cup over medium heat just until the beeswax is melted. Remove from the heat.

2. Stir in the rose wax, to melt. Continue stirring until the rose wax is incorporated into the jojoba oil–beeswax mixture. Add essential oils a few drops at a time until the fragrance is pleasing.

3. Pour into a ½-ounce tin. Label and date.

TO USE

Apply to pulse points.

✳ Frankincense and Coconut Oil Deodorant

Natural deodorants control odor but don't stop you from sweating. Commercial deodorants contain carcinogens, endocrine disruptors, and toxins. Using a natural deodorant after years of using commercial deodorants will cause your body to excrete the toxins. You may experience a rash or you may temporarily have an increase in body odor. If you 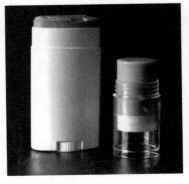 develop a rash, discontinue using the natural product for three or four days, or until the rash stops. Then you can begin to use it again.

This wax-based deodorant has some clay to encourage the detoxification process, while myrrh and frankincense stop odor with their antimicrobial actions.

YIELD: 1 (4-ounce) container

INGREDIENTS

2 tablespoons beeswax

2 tablespoons cocoa butter

3 tablespoons coconut oil

1 tablespoon baking soda

2 tablespoons kaolin clay

¼ teaspoon frankincense essential oil

¼ teaspoon myrrh essential oil

25 drops cedar atlas essential oil

DIRECTIONS

1. Create a double boiler using a glass measuring cup. Simmer the beeswax, cocoa butter, and coconut oil in the measuring cup just until the beeswax melts.

2. Stir together to incorporate the wax and the oils. Remove from the heat. Stir in the baking soda and clay, beating together with a whisk to fully incorporate. Continue to stir while the mixture cools somewhat.

3. When it is warm enough to touch the side of the dish and mixture just begins to thicken, stir in the essential oils.

4. Spoon into a push-up deodorant container. Allow this to harden fully before using. Label and date.

While the product looks dark because of the clay, it won't darken your skin. It doesn't feel greasy or waxy. Use as you would any deodorant.

🐝 Lemon-Chamomile Cuticle Butter

Massage this cuticle butter into your fingers and nail beds several times a day to heal dry and damaged skin, hang nails, and weather-damaged hands. Chamomile flowers calm inflamed skin. The jojoba oil is a natural wax that allows the infused oils to go deeper into the nail bed. The more you use it, the more beneficial the effects will be. Sunflower oil is one of the best oils for healing damaged skin.

YIELD: 1 (2-ounce) tube

INGREDIENTS

1 tablespoon jojoba oil

2 tablespoons sunflower oil

½ teaspoon lanolin

1 teaspoon mango butter

2 teaspoons dried chamomile flowers

1 tablespoon beeswax pastilles

¼ teaspoon vitamin E oil

25 drops chamomile essential oil

10 drops lemon verbena essential oil

DIRECTIONS

1. Create a double boiler using a glass measuring cup. Add jojoba oil, sunflower oil, lanolin, and mango butter to the cup. Place the loose chamomile flowers in a paper tea bag, and place the tea bag in the measuring cup with the oils. Simmer on medium heat for one hour. Turn off the heat and let the infused oil come to room temperature naturally. Remove the tea bag and press it between two spoons over the cup to get as much oil as possible from it. Discard the tea bag.

2. Add the beeswax to the measuring cup. Return the saucepan to the heat. Simmer over low heat just long enough to melt the beeswax.

3. Remove from the heat. Whisk the butter together while it cools to keep the texture creamy. When it is just warm to the touch, stir in the vitamin E and essential oils.

4. Pour into a push-up tube. Label and date.

TO USE

Rub into nails and cuticles to moisturize and protect. The more often you use this the more beneficial it will be.

🐝 Nail Conditioner

Nail and cuticle conditioner protects the nails from absorbing too much water while at the same time sealing in natural oils. Regular use can strengthen nails and heal skin that is cracked and dry from gardening or cleaning. Package this in a purse-size tube so that you can carry it with you to massage on during the in-between moments: waiting for the bus, standing in line, or sitting in the parking lot.

YIELD: 2 (1-ounce) push-up tubes

INGREDIENTS

1 tablespoon beeswax

1 tablespoon avocado butter

1 tablespoon calendula-infused olive oil

1 tablespoon argan oil

¼ teaspoon vitamin E oil

10 drops lavender essential oil

10 drops tea tree essential oil

DIRECTIONS

1. Create a double boiler using a glass measuring cup. Simmer the beeswax, avocado butter, calendula-infused olive oil, and argan oil in the cup on medium heat just long enough to melt the beeswax. Remove from the heat.

2. Whisk the butter together while it cools to keep the texture creamy. When it is just warm to the touch, stir in the vitamin E and essential oils.

3. Spoon into push-up containers for ease of use. Label and date.

TO USE

Rub into nails and cuticles to moisturize and protect. The more often you use this, the more beneficial it will be.

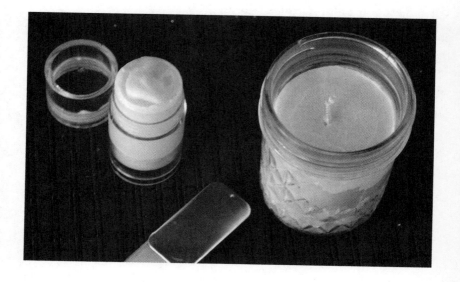

Massage Products

Massage can be therapeutic, comforting, or intimate. Beeswax, body butters, and oils reduce the friction and increase warmth and relaxation. Herb-infused oils can increase the therapeutic benefits of massage while increasing lymph flow and reducing pain and inflammation. Aromatherapy, through the use of essential oils, can heighten relaxation.

🌟 Chocolate Massage Truffles

These truffles aren't for eating. They are for pain relief, relaxation, and comfort. With the heady fragrance of chocolate, they are served up in single serving sizes. Mold them in a silicone chocolate mold for best effect. They make a lovely gift.

YIELD: 24 (1½-teaspoon) servings

INGREDIENTS

3 tablespoons cocoa butter

4 tablespoons beeswax

2 tablespoons St. John's wort–infused oil

1 tablespoon Balm of Gilead–infused oil

3 tablespoons melted coconut oil

¼ teaspoon vitamin E oil

5 drops frankincense essential oil

5 drops cinnamon essential oil

1 drop myrrh essential oil

1 drop vetiver essential oil

DIRECTIONS

1. Make a double boiler using a glass measuring cup. Simmer the cocoa butter, beeswax, infused oils, and coconut oil in the cup until your cocoa butter, beeswax, and oils melt. You won't need to boil the water; steaming it is enough. Once the beeswax

mixture is melted, remove from the heat. Stir well as the mixture cools.

2. When the mixture begins to cool and thicken, stir in the vitamin E and the essential oils. Pour about 1½ teaspoons into each mold indentation.

3. Cool completely to room temperature. Pop out of the molds. Store in a glass jar in a cool, dry place. Label and date.

TO USE

Melt the massage truffle between warm hands and use the rich oil to massage into the back and body. Continue the massage until the oils are fully absorbed into the body and the skin is dry, about 15 minutes.

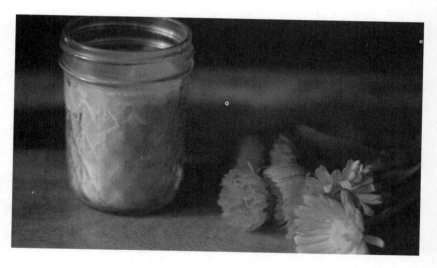

✳ Massage Candle

Massage candles combine the warmth of melted wax therapy with massage, skin care, and aromatherapy. They make lovely and unusual gifts.

YIELD: 1 (4-ounce) candle

INGREDIENTS

4 tablespoons beeswax

4 tablespoons shea butter

2 teaspoons pine resin

3 tablespoons coconut oil

1 tablespoon avocado butter

25 drops spruce or pine essential oil

25 drops frankincense essential oil

20 drops rosemary essential oil

EQUIPMENT

1 4-ounce jar or other fire-safe container

Prepared candle wick in tab

Bobby pin

2 bamboo skewers

DIRECTIONS

1. Make a double boiler using a glass measuring cup. Melt together the beeswax, shea butter, pine resin, coconut oil, and avocado butter in the cup. Stir while it is melting so that the pine doesn't end up on the bottom of the container.

2. Prepare the jar. Dip the candle wick tab in melted wax. Insert the tab into the jar and press down in the center of the bottom of the jar to secure it in place. Insert the end of the wick through the hole in a bobby pin. Turn the bobby pin so that it is perpendicular to the wick. Lay bamboo skewers, one on either side of the wick, on the rim of the jar, to hold the wick in the center of the jar. Set aside.

3. When the wax and butters have melted, remove from the heat. Stir to completely combine the pine resin with the wax, butter, and oil. Add the essential oils.

4. Pour into the mold, keeping the wick centered. Stop pouring within one-half inch of the top of the jar.

5. Allow the candle wax to cool naturally. The candle will cool in the center last. Fill the hollow around the wick with additional melted wax mixture as necessary to make the top of the candle level.

TO USE

1. Light the wick and burn the candle long enough to create a small pool of wax.

2. Blow out the flame. Allow the wax to cool slightly. You don't want the wax to be too hot.

3. Test the wax to make sure it's not too hot. Pour or scoop the soft wax mixture out of the candle and apply the warm wax mixture directly to the skin.

4. Use it as part of a massage with additional massage oil, or use it alone. Burn as much or as little of the candle as you want to. Any wax that you don't use will harden and can be used next time.

Warm wax massage is deeply relaxing and therapeutic.

Up until now, the recipes in this book have focused on oil- and wax-based mixtures that take advantage of beeswax's texturizing and protecting properties. **Emulsified lotions and creams** are an entirely different category of skin care.

Like Galen's Cold Cream, skin care lotions or creams feel wonderfully hydrating on your skin because of the high percentage of water-based ingredients in them. Lotions or creams are mixtures of oil and water held in contact with the addition of an emulsifier. You know when you make a vinaigrette salad dressing, how the oil sits on top of the vinegar? You need to shake it a lot to blend the oil and vinegar before pouring. But it doesn't matter how long you shake it for. Within a few minutes, the oil and vinegar will separate again, unless you add an emulsifier, like mustard or eggs.

When trying to make a lotion with beeswax, you need a 50/50 blend of oil- and water-based ingredients. If you put too many water-based ingredients into the recipe, your oil and beeswax will float on top of your product rather than staying mixed. Emulsifiers help in mixing beeswax and oil mixtures with water-based ingredients. Beeswax alone is not a complete emulsifier, but when combined with borax, beeswax creates a chemical reaction, which allows oil and water to emulsify. The addition of liquid lecithin can encourage the beeswax and borax emulsion to remain stable.

When making a lotion or cream with beeswax, borax, and lecithin, the oil portion of the mixture will be equal to the water portion. The combination of beeswax, borax, and lecithin is not as strong an emulsifier as synthetic emulsifying wax. You cannot take a recipe that uses emulsifying wax and substitute beeswax, borax, and lecithin for the emulsifying wax called for in the recipe. Each type of emulsifying wax has its own unique requirements.

When water is added to any beauty product, the environment is right for microbes to reproduce. The introduction of water-based ingredients sets up the mixture for microbial growth. Make small batches of lotions and creams and plan to use them up, or refrigerate them for longer term storage. How long the cream will last in your fridge is affected by several factors. Some lotions may become moldy within three weeks, while other lotions may last six months. However, the shelf life can be extended with the addition of a germicide. Follow the manufacturer's directions for using any germicidal product. The directions vary according to the brand used. (See Resources on page 278.)

Here are some tips for making lotions and creams:

* Work in a clean and sanitized work space.

* Use stainless steel or glass equipment, and sterilize it before proceeding.

* Use distilled, boiled, or bottled water. Do not use tap water or spring water.

* Use dried herbs and botanicals, never fresh.

* Heat the oil phase separately to 160°F. Heat the water phase just until it's warm enough to dissolve the borax. Then, allow both to cool to 90°F. Add the essential oils and vitamin E to the oil phase before blending.

* Add the water to the oil, not the other way around.

* As you combine the oil and water phases, mix with an immersion blender to completely blend it.

* When blending with an immersion blender, use a container that allows the blender to remain under the surface of the mixture to avoid adding air to the mixture.

* Pour the mixture into a clean, sterilized jar before it has cooled completely. It will continue to firm up as it cools.

* To avoid condensation on the underside of the caps, do not place a lid on the jars until they are completely cool. Wipe the inside of the caps with alcohol before packaging the product.

* Keep the product refrigerated unless you add a germicide.

🐝 Rose Silk Facial Cream

This lotion is hydrating and full of the rich scent of roses from both the rose hydrosol and the rose wax.

YIELD: 2 (2-ounce) jars

INGREDIENTS

Oil Phase

1 tablespoon beeswax

1 teaspoon rose wax

2 tablespoons mango butter

1 teaspoon liquid sunflower lecithin

2 tablespoons rose-infused olive oil

Water Phase

5 tablespoons rose hydrosol

1 teaspoon silk protein powder

¼ teaspoon borax

10 drops rose absolute or rose geranium essential oil

DIRECTIONS

1. Make a double boiler using a 2-cup glass measuring cup. Simmer the beeswax, rose wax, mango butter, sunflower lecithin, and olive oil in the cup over low heat until the oil and wax reaches 155°F or until the beeswax is fully melted. Remove from the heat.

2. In a second glass measuring cup, combine the rose hydrosol, silk protein powder, and borax. Place in a second saucepan with water and heat just until the borax dissolves.

3. Stir the beeswax oil mixture while it is cooling to prevent it from forming clumps. Add the essential oil to the oil mixture. When the oil mixture reaches about 90°F and the water is also at 90°F, begin blending the oil portion with an immersion blender. Slowly drizzle the hydrosol-borax mixture into the oils a few drops at a time, while blending the mixture.

4. The mixture will become white and creamy. Continue blending until all the hydrosol mixture is incorporated into the wax-oil mixture and the emulsion is complete. This will take about 5 to 10 minutes of blending.

5. Spoon this mixture into jars. Label and date. Since this recipe does not contain a preservative, keep the jars in the fridge when not in use. If you see any signs of spoilage, discard and make a fresh batch.

TO USE

Use this fragrant moisturizer as a daytime facial cream. It is lighter and more fragrant than oil-based lotion bars. It may still feel greasy to those who are accustomed to commercial lotions. You can prolong the shelf life by incorporating a broad spectrum antimicrobial into the water phase before blending the two phases of the lotion together. Follow the manufacturer's instructions.

🐝 Galen's Cold Cream

In my younger years, I clowned around and performed as a mime. I used this cold cream to remove the white and grease makeup after a day of making animal twisty balloons at a children's hospital. This is one of the oldest cosmetic recipes known. It was developed by the Greek physician Galen (CE 150). The original recipe called for olive oil infused with rose petals and rose water. If you have rose petal–infused olive oil, go ahead and substitute that for the olive oil in this recipe.

YIELD: 1 (4-ounce) jar

INGREDIENTS

Oil Phase

1 tablespoon beeswax

¼ teaspoon sunflower lecithin

3 tablespoons olive oil

Water Phase

¼ teaspoon borax

3 tablespoons rose hydrosol

DIRECTIONS

1. Make a double boiler using a glass measuring cup. Simmer the beeswax, sunflower lecithin, and olive oil in the cup over low heat until the oil and wax reaches 155°F or until the beeswax is fully melted. Remove from the heat.

2. In a second glass measuring cup, combine the borax and rose hydrosol. Place in a second saucepan with water and heat just until the borax dissolves.

3. Stir the beeswax oil mixture while it is cooling to prevent it from forming clumps. When the oil mixture reaches about 90°F and

the water is also at 90°F, begin blending the oil portion with an immersion blender. Slowly drizzle the hydrosol–borax mixture into the oils a few drops at a time, while continuing to blend.

4. The mixture will become white and creamy. Continue blending until all the hydrosol mixture is incorporated into the wax-oil mixture and the emulsion is complete. This will take about 5 to 10 minutes.

5. Spoon this mixture into a 4-ounce jar. Label and date. Since this recipe does not contain a preservative, keep the jar in the fridge when not in use. If you see any signs of spoilage, discard it and make a fresh batch.

TO USE

Rub a small amount onto the face. Use a tissue to remove the excess. It will remove makeup and dirt as the excess is wiped off.

Chapter 4

BEESWAX IN SOAP AND HAIR CARE

What soap is to the body, laughter is to the soul.

—Yiddish proverb

Playing with beeswax is often a gateway to more self-reliance, a moving away from dependence on multinational corporations to meet our daily needs. Those who play with beeswax shift into a greater sense of responsibility for self, for family, and for the earth. It may begin with a lip balm recipe or a few candles, and before you know it, you are comfortable making your own soap, shampoo, and hair care items, just like families did in the centuries before us.

Making soap was a milestone for me in the do-it-yourself journey. The first time I made soap it was magical. Taking liquid oils and lye and mixing them together creates a chemical reaction that produces heat and transforms oil or fats, which are extremely hard to clean up, into something that actually enables other things to be cleaned.

Handmade soap contains moisturizing glycerin, a by-product of soap making. Commercially, this glycerin is removed from the soap because it's worth more when sold separately than when left in the soap. Handmade soap has all this valuable glycerin incorporated into the lather, ready to soothe and moisturize your skin.

All soap is made with lye. But properly-made soap contains no lye. All lye used in the soapmaking process is converted to soap through the chemical process of saponification.

Lots of people are intimidated by soapmaking. They are afraid of the lye, and rightly so. Lye is a caustic chemical that can cause very bad burns. But when treated with respect, lye can transform fats and oils into a valuable and coveted product. Soapmaking is a foundational skill in the do-it-yourself repertoire.

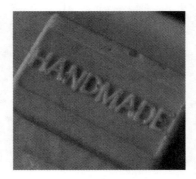

Lye Safety

Before I talk to you about beeswax and soap, let's begin by talking about lye safety. While I want you to respect lye, I don't want you to be afraid of it. Lye, or sodium hydroxide, is caustic. When you add powdered lye to a liquid, the lye dissolves and the liquid heats up. It gets hot enough to boil and splash, and that splash is no longer water but liquid lye. It can be made from sweat from your hands, a drop of water on the counter, or the water in your mixing bowl.

Always add lye to liquid, never liquid to lye. By adding the lye to the water, you can control the reaction and keep it in the bowl. Lye is highly alkaline. Keep a jug of white vinegar nearby, because vinegar buffers the caustic reaction of the lye.

Wear protective goggles when you are working with lye, and chemical-resistant gloves that cover your wrists and forearms. Disposable latex gloves do not offer enough protection against lye burns. Normal latex cleaning gloves will warp from the heat of the lye and could allow some lye through. So use chemical-resistant gloves when you are working with the lye powder and the liquid lye. You can safely switch to latex gloves once the lye is incorporated into the fat.

When you add the lye to the liquid, caustic vapors are released. Work in a well-ventilated area. Avert your face from the fumes. I set up a fan to carry the fumes outside through an open window. My husband prefers to make soap on an outdoor porch. Do not make soap with young children or pets in the room.

If you accidentally splash lye on yourself, splash the area immediately with vinegar to neutralize the alkalinity, and then flush with tap water until there is no burning sensation. If you splash lye in your face or in your eyes, immediately flush your face and eyes with cold water, and go to the hospital emergency room for treatment. They have an eye bath for chemical burns. After all that warning, let me say that I have never had a serious burn from lye in thirty-plus years of soapmaking. You need to take sensible precautions in soapmaking, but don't be fearful.

A fellow farmer's market vendor told me a story of when he and his brother made soap for the first time. They were drinking beer at the same time. When they got to the point where the soap was at "trace" and looked creamy and rich like vanilla pudding, they lifted the spoon to their mouths to have a taste. Don't be these men. Green soap is not yet fully saponified and the soap can burn, like lye. They learned their lesson the hard way. Don't drink and saponify.

The Value of Beeswax in Soapmaking

Beeswax can be a useful ingredient in handmade soap. Beeswax makes handmade soap bars harder and last longer. It also makes soap milder and increases the moisturizing effect of soap. Beeswax should only take up 5 percent to 8 percent of your recipe. If you add too much, you will reduce the amount and quality of the lather. Also, too much beeswax combined with hard oils like shea butter or cocoa butter can cause the bar of soap to crack as it cools.

Different oils and fats require different amounts of lye to turn them from fats into soap using a chemical process called saponification.

The amount of lye needed for this process is called the saponification value. It is relevant only when you reformulate a soap recipe or develop your own soap recipes. Beeswax saponifies with the oil ingredients in a soap recipe and must be included in the lye calculation. Its saponification value is 88 to 100. Please refer to an online lye calculator when formulating your own recipes or when substituting any of the ingredients in the soap recipes in this book. See Resources on page 278.

Beeswax melts at 140°F to 147°F, which is hotter than the melting point for your other oils, so melt the beeswax separately and add it to your other oils after they are melted.

Soap recipes are calculated by weight instead of volume, with the exception of the liquid used to dissolve the lye and any essential oils or other additives that are added at the end of the recipe. Please use a scale and take the time to measure accurately to ensure success. The lye must be weighed accurately so that all the lye in the recipe is saponified with the fat. If too much lye is used in relationship to the fats and oils, there will be unsaponified lye in the soap, and the soap will be harsh and drying.

The recipes in this book make approximately 3 pounds of soap, or 12 4-ounce bars.

What Is Trace?

Trace is the point in the soapmaking process when the oils and lye solution have emulsified. The oils are no longer separated in the mixture but are integrated. The mixture becomes thick like pudding. At trace, a trailing of the soap will sit on the surface of the soap mixture without sinking back in immediately. It is at trace that the soap additives like essential oils are added to the soap.

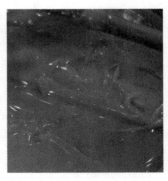

Soap at trace

Equipment for Soapmaking

All utensils and equipment used for soapmaking should be made of nonreactive stainless steel, glass, or silicone. Although wooden utensils can be used, lye will damage wooden spoons.

There are a few pieces of equipment you'll use every time you make soap.

* 2-cup glass measuring cup
* 4-cup glass measuring cup
* Digital scale
* Glass rod or silicone spatula
* Immersion blender
* Saucepan for double boiler
* Soap mold with 3-pound (48-fluid-ounce) capacity
* Spatula
* Stainless steel pot

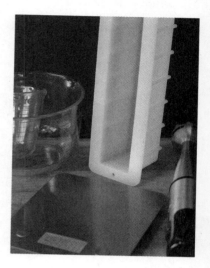

Soap Molds

The recipes in this book make a three-pound batch of soap. Soap molds need to be prepared before you mix the lye solution with the oils. Silicone and plastic molds used for soap making should be sprayed with silicone mold release to make it easier to remove the soap from the mold. Wooden or cardboard molds should be lined with parchment paper to prepare the molds for soapmaking. Silicone, plastic, and cardboard molds are flimsy and will need to be supported by a board or tray when they are filled with liquid soap. Wooden molds are stable and can be used without extra support.

Any surface that the soap mold is placed on should be protected from excessive heat. The soap mixture may heat up in the first 48 hours after it is made. This is part of the saponification process.

🐝 Basic Beeswax Soap

This is a practice bar of soap to help you master the technique of making cold-processed soap. Follow the recipe carefully.

YIELD: 12 (4-ounce) bars

INGREDIENTS

5½ ounces lye (NaOH)

14 fluid ounces water

18 ounces coconut oil

18 ounces olive oil

2 ounces beeswax

1 to 2 teaspoons essential oil of your choice

DIRECTIONS

1. Choose a well-ventilated area to work. While wearing safety goggles and gloves, weigh the lye. Pour the lye into the water in a 4-cup glass measuring cup while stirring to fully dissolve the lye. Set aside and allow this to cool to 105°F to 120°F. Avert your face from the dissolving lye. Do not breathe in the lye fumes.

2. Combine the coconut oil and olive oil in a 6-quart stainless steel stock pot and heat gently to 150°F. Remove from the heat.

3. Place the beeswax in a glass measuring cup, inside a saucepan. Fill the saucepan with 3 inches of water. Simmer just until the beeswax is melted. Remove from the heat.

4. Pour a small amount of the warmed oils into the melted beeswax, stirring to keep the beeswax from hardening. Continue adding warmed oil keeping the beeswax mixture liquid. Transfer all the beeswax mixture to the warmed oil and stir well to fully incorporate. Allow this to cool to 105°F to 125°F.

5. While the lye solution and the oil-wax mixture are cooling, prepare your soap molds. Silicone molds need to be supported by a tray. Wooden molds need to be lined with parchment paper.

Cardboard molds should be lined with plastic wrap, and the whole mold should be supported with a firm tray. This will make the soap easier to unmold when the bars are done.

6. When the lye solution and the oil mixture cool to within the correct temperature range, pour the lye mixture into the oil mixture, being careful not to splash the lye while combining. Stir the mixture using an immersion blender. Beeswax speeds up the saponification process, so you may find that trace happens more quickly in beeswax soap.

7. Continue stirring the soap mixture until it traces. At trace, if you pull the immersion blender out of the mixture and let it drip on the surface of the pot, the mixture will support the drip, instead of allowing it to immediately settle back into the vat.

8. Once trace occurs, add in any essential oils that you want. Good essential oil choices are lavender, lemon, sweet orange, bergamot, peppermint, or tea tree. Use any combination that smells good to you, adding a total of 1 to 2 teaspoons of essential oils. Use 2 teaspoons if using citrus oils and 1 teaspoon for other oils like peppermint or lavender.

9. Mix the essential oils into the soap. Continue stirring until the soap has the consistency of lemon curd or chilled pudding. Pour the soap into the mold. Smooth the surface of the soap in the mold using a silicone spatula.

10. Cover the top of the mold with a board to hold in the heat. Cover all of this with a towel. Set the soap aside to complete the saponification process. The soap will go through a gel phase where the temperature of the soap rises, making it translucent. Then, as the saponification finishes, the soap will become opaque and firm. During this process, protect the surface underneath the mold from excessive heat. After 24 to 48 hours, the soap should be completely opaque with no translucent areas. At this time, the soap can be removed from the mold. The saponification process is almost done. It will continue inside the finished bar of soap for up to three weeks after the soap is made. Wearing

gloves, cut the soap into twelve 4-ounce bars. Stack the bars on a nonreactive tray to dry. Set aside for three weeks.

11. After three weeks, package the soap. It is now ready to use, but the soap will improve with age, like fine wine. Soap has no expiry date.

🐝 Honey Soap

This is the beekeeper's soap, rich in moisturizers, mild, and gentle to the skin. Honey is a humectant, attracting water to itself, while beeswax prevents moisture loss. The combination results in a super-moisturizing soap. If you are a beekeeper, keep the bar unscented so that you don't upset your bees with foreign scents. For everyone else, enjoy a mild fragranced soap, like lemongrass.

Adding honey or any kind of sugar to soap is an advanced soapmaking technique. If you are new to soapmaking, try the basic bar first before attempting this soap. Honey causes the soap to heat up more during the gel phase, which can damage the texture of the soap. To improve the texture, this soap is prevented from going through the gel phase by being placed in the freezer for a full 24 hours.

YIELD: 12 (4-ounce) bars

INGREDIENTS

4½ ounces lye (NaOH)

14 fluid ounces water

10 ounces coconut oil

10 ounces olive oil

8 ounces jojoba oil

4 ounces castor oil

4 ounces shea butter

2 ounces beeswax

2 tablespoons honey

1 teaspoon lemon-grass essential oil (optional)

DIRECTIONS

1. Choose a well-ventilated area to work. While wearing safety goggles and gloves, weigh the lye. Pour the lye into the water in a four cup glass measuring cup while stirring to fully dissolve the lye. Set aside and allow this to cool to 105°F to 120°F. Avert your face from the dissolving lye. Do not breathe in the lye fumes.

2. Combine the coconut oil, olive oil, jojoba oil, castor oil, and shea butter in a 6-quart stainless steel stock pot and heat gently to 150°F. Remove from the heat.

3. Place the beeswax in a glass measuring cup, inside a saucepan. Fill the saucepan with 3 inches of water. Simmer just until the beeswax is melted. Remove from the heat.

4. Pour a small amount of the warmed oils into the melted beeswax while stirring to keep the beeswax from hardening. Continue adding warmed oil keeping the beeswax mixture liquid. Transfer all the beeswax mixture to the warmed oil and stir well to fully incorporate. Allow this to cool to 105°F to 125°F.

5. While the lye solution and the oil-wax mixture are cooling, prepare your soap molds. Put the honey in a separate glass measuring cup and place the measuring cup in a bowl of warm water to allow the honey to be poured more easily.

6. When the lye solution and the oil-wax mixture cool to within the correct temperature range, pour the lye mixture into the oil mixture, being careful not to splash the lye while combining. Stir the mixture using an immersion blender. Beeswax speeds up the saponification process, so you may find that trace happens more quickly in beeswax soap.

7. Continue stirring the soap mixture until it traces. At trace, if you pull the immersion blender out of the mixture and let it drip on the surface of the pot, the mixture will support the drip instead of allowing it to immediately settle back into the vat. Once trace occurs, add the warmed honey and essential oil

to the soap mixture. Continue stirring until the soap has the consistency of lemon curd or chilled pudding, and the honey and essential oil are fully incorporated.

8. Pour the soap mixture into prepared molds. Smooth the surface of the soap using a silicone spatula. Place the soap molds onto a baking sheet. Cover the molds with plastic wrap. Place the baking sheet with the molds into the freezer in order to prevent the soap from going through the gel phase of saponification. The soap must remain in the freezer for a full 24 hours. The soap is finished saponifying when it is cold to the touch, with no warm places.

9. Remove the soap from the freezer. Allow the soap to return to room temperature before you cut it into bars. If there is condensation, wipe it off with a paper towel. Wearing gloves, cut the soap into 12 4-ounce bars. Allow it to air dry. Stack the bars on a nonreactive tray to dry. Set aside for three weeks.

10. After three weeks, package the soap. It is now ready to use, but the soap will improve with age, like fine wine. Soap has no expiry date.

🐝 Mechanic's Hand Soap

Sweet orange oil helps remove the grease and grime from your hands, without the harsh abrasives found in commercial hand cleaners. The inherent moisturizers will help keep your skin supple and prevent it from drying out.

YIELD: 12 (4-ounce) bars

INGREDIENTS

5.2 ounces lye (NaOH)

14 fluid ounces water

10 ounces coconut oil

10 ounces olive oil

10 ounces hemp seed oil

3 ounces castor oil

3 ounces cocoa butter

2 ounces beeswax

1 tablespoon d-limonene

1 teaspoon sweet orange essential oil

5 tablespoons freshly ground coffee

4 tablespoons ground walnut shells (optional; omit if allergic to nuts)

DIRECTIONS

1. Choose a well-ventilated area to work. While wearing safety goggles and gloves, weigh the lye. Pour the lye into the water in a 4-cup glass measuring cup while stirring to fully dissolve the lye. Set aside and allow this to cool to 105°F to 120°F. Avert your face from the dissolving lye. Do not breathe in the lye fumes.

2. Combine the coconut oil, olive oil, hemp seed oil, castor oil, and cocoa butter in a 6-quart stainless steel stock pot and heat gently to 150°F. Remove from the heat.

3. Place the beeswax in a glass measuring cup, inside a saucepan. Fill the saucepan with 3 inches of water. Simmer just until the beeswax is melted. Remove from the heat.

4. Pour a small amount of the warmed oils into the melted beeswax while stirring to keep the beeswax from hardening. Continue adding warmed oil to the beeswax mixture to keep the beeswax mixture liquid. Transfer all the beeswax mixture to the warmed oil and stir well to fully incorporate. Allow this to cool to 105°F to 125°F.

5. While the lye solution and the oil-wax mixture are cooling, prepare your soap molds. Silicone molds need to be supported by a tray. Wooden molds need to be lined with parchment paper. Cardboard molds should be lined with plastic wrap, and the whole mold should be supported with a firm tray. This will make the soap easier to unmold when the bars are done.

6. When the lye solution and the oil–wax mixture cool to within the correct temperature range, pour the lye mixture into the oil mixture, being careful not to splash the lye while combining. Stir the mixture using an immersion blender. Beeswax speeds up the saponification process, so you may find that trace happens more quickly in beeswax soap.

7. Continue stirring the soap mixture until it traces. At trace, if you pull the immersion blender out of the mixture and let it drip on the surface of the pot, the mixture will support the drip instead of allowing it to immediately settle back into the vat. Once trace occurs, add the d–limonene, sweet orange essential oil, ground coffee, and ground walnut shells, if using. Continue stirring until the soap has thickened like lemon curd or chilled pudding. It will be grainy.

8. Pour the soap into the prepared mold. Smooth the surface of the soap in the mold.

9. Cover the top of the mold with a board to hold in the heat. Cover all of this with a towel. Set the soap aside to complete the saponification process. The soap will go through a gel phase where the temperature of the soap rises, making it translucent. Then, as the saponification finishes, the soap will become opaque and firm. During this process, protect the surface underneath the mold from excessive heat.

10. After 24 to 48 hours, the soap should be completely opaque, with no translucent areas. The soap can be removed from the mold. The saponification process is almost done. It will continue inside the finished bars of soap for up to three weeks after the soap is made. Wearing gloves, cut the soap into twelve 4–ounce bars. Stack the bars on a nonreactive tray to dry. Set aside for three weeks.

11. After three weeks, package the soap. It is now ready to use, but the soap will improve with age. Soap has no expiry date.

🦟 Gardener's Soap

Gardeners benefit from a mild soap with a gentle abrasiveness and rich moisturizing qualities. Cuticles and nails are especially punished during gardening season, with planting, weeding, and harvesting. This super-fatted recipe will protect your hands, even with frequent hand washing.

YIELD: 12 (4-ounce) bars

INGREDIENTS

5.1 ounces lye (NaOH)

14 fluid ounces water

10 ounces coconut oil

10 ounces olive oil

4 ounces castor oil

4 ounces mango butter

8 ounces cocoa butter

2 ounces beeswax

1 teaspoon lemon essential oil

1 teaspoon eucalyptus essential oil

½ teaspoon tea tree essential oil

1 tablespoon dried, ground orange peel

2 tablespoons whole poppy seeds

DIRECTIONS

1. Choose a well-ventilated area to work. While wearing safety goggles and gloves, weigh the lye. Pour the lye into the water in a 4-cup glass measuring cup while stirring to fully dissolve the lye. Set aside and allow this to cool to 105°F to 120°F. Avert your face from the dissolving lye. Do not breathe in the lye fumes.

2. Combine the coconut oil, olive oil, castor oil, mango butter, and cocoa butter in a 6-quart stainless steel stock pot and heat gently to 150°F. Remove from the heat.

3. Place the beeswax in a glass measuring cup, inside a saucepan. Fill the saucepan with 3 inches of water. Simmer just until the beeswax is melted. Remove from the heat.

4. Pour a small amount of the warmed oils into the melted beeswax while stirring to keep the beeswax from hardening. Continue adding warmed oil to keep the beeswax mixture liquid. Transfer the beeswax mixture to the warmed oil and stir well to fully incorporate. Allow this to cool to 105°F to 125°F.

5. While the lye solution and the oil-wax mixture are cooling, prepare your soap molds. Silicone molds need to be supported by a tray. Wooden molds need to be lined with parchment paper. Cardboard molds should be lined with plastic wrap, and the whole mold should be supported with a firm tray. This will make the soap easier to unmold when the bars are done.

6. When the lye solution and the oil-wax mixture cool to the correct temperature ranges, pour the lye mixture into the oil mixture, being careful not to splash the lye while combining. Stir the mixture using an immersion blender. Beeswax speeds up the saponification process, so you may find that trace happens more quickly in beeswax soap.

7. Continue stirring the soap mixture until it traces. At trace, if you pull the immersion blender out of the mixture and let it drip on the surface of the pot, the mixture will support the drip instead of allowing it to immediately settle back into the vat. Once trace occurs, add in the essential oils, ground orange peel, and poppy seeds. Continue stirring until the soap has thickened like lemon curd or chilled pudding.

8. Pour the soap into the mold. Smooth the surface of the soap in the mold.

9. Cover the top of the mold with a board to hold in the heat. Cover all of this with a towel. Set the soap aside to complete the saponification process. The soap will go through a gel phase where the temperature of the soap rises, making it translucent. Then, as the saponification finishes, the soap will become opaque and firm. During this process, protect the surface underneath the mold from excessive heat.

10. After 24 to 48 hours, the soap should be completely opaque, with no translucent areas. The soap can be removed from the mold. The saponification process is almost done. It will continue inside the finished bars of soap for up to three weeks after the soap is made. Wearing gloves, cut the soap into twelve 4-ounce bars. Stack the bars on a nonreactive tray to dry. Set aside for three weeks.

11. After three weeks, package the soap. It is now ready to use, but the soap will improve with age, like fine wine. Soap has no expiry date.

Hair care: Commercial shampoo damages hair, strips it of its natural oils, and causes denaturing of the protein in the hair shaft. Many opt for "no-poo," using baking soda and vinegar to clean their hair. But baking soda can be harsh and messy, and the no-poo method is a little inconvenient when you are traveling. These shampoo bars consist of real, natural soap, rich in moisturizers for your hair, with rich lather and built-in conditioners.

As an added bonus, when traveling, shampoo bars can be packed in your carry-on luggage and do not contribute to your liquid allowance during security checks.

When using a natural shampoo, it's important to restore your hair's natural pH balance by using a vinegar rinse after the final shampoo. In this chapter I've included a recipe for my favorite vinegar hair rinses, which encourage natural hair color highlights.

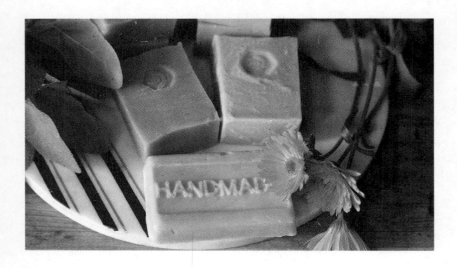

✳ Infused Vinegar Rinse for Fair Hair

YIELD: 3 cups (about 24 applications)

INGREDIENTS

3 cups cider or white vinegar

1 cup dried chamomile blossoms

¼ cup dried lemon peel

DIRECTIONS

1. Simmer vinegar, chamomile blossoms, and lemon peel in a pot over low heat for 30 minutes. Turn off the heat. Allow the pot to cool naturally.

2. Press out the plant material. Reserve the liquid.

TO USE

Place 2 tablespoons of the infused vinegar in 1 cup of lukewarm water. Rinse hair after shampooing. Pour over hair. Rinse again. Dry hair as usual.

🐝 Infused Vinegar Rinse for Dark Hair

YIELD: 3 cups (about 24 applications)

INGREDIENTS

3 cups cider or white vinegar

1 cup dried rosemary leaves

¼ cup dried sage leaves

DIRECTIONS

1. Simmer vinegar, rosemary, and sage in a pot over low heat for 30 minutes. Turn off the heat. Allow the pot to cool naturally.

2. Press out the plant material. Reserve the liquid.

TO USE

Place 2 tablespoons of the infused vinegar in 1 cup of lukewarm water. Rinse hair after shampooing. Pour over hair. Rinse again. Dry hair as usual.

🐝 Chamomile Shampoo Bars for Fair Hair

This is a gentle shampoo that works for naturally fair hair and bleached or damaged hair. It's gentle on the hair and contains no SLS or harsh chemicals. Argan oil is rich in fatty acids and vitamin E for conditioning your hair as you shampoo.

YIELD: 12 (4-ounce) bars

INGREDIENTS

2 cups water

1 ounce dried chamomile flowers

4.85 ounces lye (NaOH)

1 teaspoon silk protein

10 ounces coconut oil

10 ounces olive oil

4 ounces argan oil

4 ounces castor oil

4 ounces jojoba oil

4 ounces mango butter

2 ounces beeswax

1 teaspoon lemon essential oil

1 teaspoon verbena essential oil

1 teaspoon cedar atlas essential oil

DIRECTIONS

1. Make strong chamomile tea by boiling 2 cups of water and pouring it over chamomile blossoms in a 4-cup glass measuring cup. Allow the tea to steep until it cools naturally. Strain out the plant material, squeezing it in a cloth to retain as much of the liquid as possible. Discard the plant material. It can be composted. Measure 14 fluid ounces of the chamomile-infused water for soapmaking, and place in a four cup glass measuring cup. The remainder can be used as a hair rinse if desired.

2. Choose a well-ventilated area to work. While wearing safety goggles and gloves, weigh the lye. Stir the lye into the room temperature, herb-infused water. Avert your face from the dissolving lye. Do not breathe in the lye fumes. Stir the silk protein into the lye mixture. Set aside to cool to 100°F to 125°F.

3. Combine the coconut oil, olive oil, argan oil, castor oil, jojoba oil, and mango butter in a 6-quart stainless steel stock pot and heat gently to 150°F. Remove from the heat.

4. Place the beeswax in a glass measuring cup, inside a saucepan. Fill the saucepan with 3 inches of water. Simmer just until the beeswax is melted. Remove from the heat.

5. Pour a small amount of the warmed oils into the melted beeswax while stirring to keep the beeswax from hardening. Continue adding warmed oil to keep the beeswax mixture liquid. Transfer all of the beeswax mixture to the warmed oil and stir well to fully incorporate. Allow this to cool to 105°F to 125°F.

6. While the lye solution and the oil-wax mixture are cooling, prepare your soap molds.

7. When the lye solution and the oil-wax mixture cool to within the correct temperature range, pour the lye mixture into the oil mixture, being careful not to splash the lye while combining. Stir the mixture using an immersion blender. Beeswax speeds up the saponification process, so you may find that trace happens more quickly in beeswax soap.

8. Continue stirring the soap mixture until it traces. At trace, if you pull the immersion blender out of the mixture and let it drip on the surface of the pot, the mixture will support the drip instead of allowing it to immediately settle back into the vat. Once trace occurs, add the essential oils. Continue stirring until the soap has the consistency of lemon curd or chilled pudding.

9. Pour the soap into the mold. Smooth the surface of the soap in the mold.

10. Cover the top of the mold with a board to hold in the heat. Cover all of this with a towel. Set the soap aside to complete the saponification process. The soap will go through a gel phase where the temperature of the soap rises, making it translucent. Then, as the saponification finishes, the soap will become opaque and firm. During this process, protect the surface underneath the mold from excessive heat. After 24 to 48 hours, the soap should be completely opaque, with no translucent areas. The soap can be removed from the mold. The saponification process is almost done. It will continue inside the finished bars of soap for up to three weeks after the soap is made. Wearing gloves, cut the soap into twelve 4-ounce bars. Stack the bars on a nonreactive tray to dry. Set aside for three weeks.

11. After three weeks, package the soap. It is now ready to use.

TO USE

1. Wet hair then rub the wet shampoo bar between your hands to work up a lather. Rub the lather into your hair and scalp. Those

with longer hair may want to rub the shampoo bar directly on their hair.

2. Massage the scalp as you would with commercial shampoo. Rinse with warm water. Repeat.

3. Follow the shampoo with the Infused Vinegar Rinse for Fair Hair (page 116) and then a rinse with plain water to restore the natural pH of the hair, which is acidic.

✳ Shampoo Bars for Dark Hair

This is a gentle shampoo that works for dark hair or damaged hair. It's gentle on hair and contains no SLS or harsh chemicals. Argan oil is rich in fatty acids and vitamin E for conditioning your hair as you shampoo. Sage and rosemary bring out dark highlights.

YIELD: 12 (4-ounce) bars

INGREDIENTS

3 cups water

1 ounce dried sage and/or rosemary leaves

4.85 ounces lye (NaOH)

1 teaspoon silk protein

10 ounces coconut oil

10 ounces olive oil

4 ounces argan oil

4 ounces castor oil

4 ounces jojoba oil

4 ounces shea butter

2 ounces beeswax

1 teaspoon rosemary essential oil

1 teaspoon thyme essential oil

1 teaspoon cedar atlas essential oil

DIRECTIONS

1. Make strong sage and rosemary tea by boiling 3 cups of water and pouring it over the leaves in a 4-cup glass measuring cup. Allow the tea to steep until it cools naturally. Strain out the plant material, squeezing it in a cloth to retain as much of the liquid as possible. Discard the plant material. It can be composted. Measure 14 fluid ounces of the sage-rosemary infused water for soapmaking in a 4-cup glass measuring cup. The remainder can be used as a hair rinse if desired.

2. Choose a well-ventilated area to work. While wearing safety goggles and gloves, weigh the lye. Stir the lye into the infused water. Avert your face from the dissolving lye. Do not breathe in the lye fumes. Stir the silk protein into the lye mixture. Set aside to cool to 100°F to 125°F.

3. Combine the coconut oil, olive oil, argan oil, castor oil, jojoba oil, and shea butter in a 6-quart stainless steel stock pot and heat gently to 150°F. Remove from the heat.

4. Place the beeswax in a glass measuring cup, inside a saucepan. Fill the saucepan with 3 inches of water. Simmer just until the beeswax is melted. Remove from the heat.

5. Pour a small amount of the warmed oils into the melted beeswax while stirring to keep the beeswax from hardening. Continue adding warmed oil keeping the beeswax mixture liquid. Transfer all the beeswax mixture to the warmed oil and stir well to fully incorporate. Allow this to cool to 105°F to 125°F.

6. While the lye solution and the oil-wax mixture are cooling, prepare your soap molds.

7. When the lye solution and the oil-wax mixture cool to within the correct temperature range, pour the lye mixture into the oil mixture, being careful not to splash the lye while combining. Stir the mixture using an immersion blender. Beeswax speeds up the saponification process, so you may find that trace happens more quickly in beeswax soap.

8. Continue stirring the soap mixture until it traces. At trace, if you pull the immersion blender out of the mixture and let it drip on the surface of the pot, the mixture will support the drip instead of allowing it to immediately settle back into the vat. Once trace occurs, add the essential oils. Continue stirring until the soap has the consistency of lemon curd or chilled pudding.

9. Pour the soap into the mold. Smooth the surface of the soap in the mold.

10. Cover the top of the mold with a board to hold in the heat. Cover all of this with a towel. Set the soap aside to complete the saponification process. The soap will go through a gel phase where the temperature of the soap rises, making it translucent. Then, as the saponification finishes, the soap will become opaque and firm. During this process, protect the surface underneath the mold from excessive heat.

11. After 24 to 48 hours, the soap should be completely opaque, with no translucent areas. The soap can be removed from the mold. The saponification process is almost done. It will continue inside the finished bars of soap for up to three weeks after the soap is made. Wearing gloves, cut the soap into twelve 4-ounce bars. Stack the bars on a nonreactive tray to dry. Set aside for three weeks.

12. After three weeks, package the soap. It is now ready to use.

TO USE

1. Wet your hair then rub the wet shampoo bar between your hands to work up a lather. Rub the lather into your hair and scalp. Those with longer hair may want to rub the shampoo bar directly on their hair.

2. Massage the scalp as you would with commercial shampoo. Rinse with warm water. Repeat.

3. Follow shampoo with the Infused Vinegar Rinse for Dark Hair (page 117) and then a rinse with plain water to restore the natural pH of the hair, which is slightly acidic.

🦟 Shaving Soap

The key to a close shave is lubrication. Many commercial shaving lubricants actually dry the skin rather than moisturize it. In order to compensate, companies add in chemical lubricants and preservatives that cause more problems. While you could use any bar soap or shampoo bar for a shaving lubricant, there isn't enough slip in normal bar soap to give you a close shave without a little blood.

Some soap makers add clay to their regular soap recipes and call the result "shaving soap." However, a properly made bar of shaving soap is rich in moisturizing butters and skin-healing oils. It will make a voluminous, lubricating lather with just a shaving brush and water.

It may seem that there are a lot of butters and oils in this bar. It's worth the extra effort. You'll definitely feel the luxury.

The choice of shaving brush is also very important to the ritual of shaving. Badger hair brushes are the best carrier for this luxurious shaving soap. It's a healthy alternative to commercial shaving foam and chemical lubricants.

Use smaller, round soap molds that will fit into a mug or a tin for this recipe. Because of the richness of the added vegetable butters, this soap has a tendency to crack on the surface as it is finishing. Using smaller molds inhibits this tendency.

YIELD: 12 (4-ounce) rounds

INGREDIENTS

3 cups water

1 ounce dried thyme

1 ounce dried rosemary

5.15 ounces lye (NaOH)

1 teaspoon silk protein

10 ounces coconut oil

4 ounces argan oil

4 ounces jojoba oil

5 ounces castor oil

3 ounces avocado butter

5 ounces mango butter

2 ounces kokum butter

2 ounces beeswax

4 teaspoons French green clay

1 teaspoon frankincense essential oil

1 teaspoon sandalwood essential oil

½ teaspoon spruce bud essential oil

½ teaspoon cedar atlas essential oil

DIRECTIONS

1. Make a strong tea with 3 cups of boiling water, rosemary, and thyme. Allow it to steep until the water cools to room temperature. Strain the tea and discard the spent herbs. Measure 14 fluid ounces of liquid into a 4-cup glass measuring cup to make your lye solution. The remainder can be used in a hair rinse, if desired.

2. Choose a well-ventilated area to work. While wearing safety goggles and gloves, weigh the lye. Stir the lye into the infused water. Avert your face from the dissolving lye. Do not breathe in the lye fumes. Stir the silk protein into the lye mixture. Set aside to cool to 100°F to 125°F.

3. Combine the coconut oil, argan oil, jojoba oil, castor oil, avocado butter, mango butter, and kokum butter in a 6-quart stainless steel stock pot and heat gently to 150°F. Stir the oils together to blend. Remove from the heat. Reserve 1 cup of the melted oils, and add the clay to this cup. Mix thoroughly to wet the clay with the oils.

4. Place the beeswax in a glass measuring cup, inside a saucepan. Fill the saucepan with 3 inches of water. Simmer just until the beeswax is melted. Remove from the heat.

5. Pour a small amount of the warmed oil into the melted beeswax while stirring to keep the beeswax from hardening. Continue adding warmed oil to keep the beeswax mixture liquid. Transfer all the beeswax mixture to the warmed oil and stir well to fully incorporate. Stir the clay-oil mixture into the oil pot as well. Allow this to cool to 105°F to 125°F.

6. While the lye solution and the oil-wax mixture are cooling, prepare your soap molds. Use silicone soap molds or hard plastic molds. Spray plastic molds with food-safe silicone spray.

7. When the lye solution and the oil-wax mixture cool to within the correct temperature range, pour the lye mixture into the oil mixture, being careful not to splash the lye while combining. Stir the mixture using an immersion blender. Beeswax speeds up the saponification process, so you may find that trace happens more quickly in beeswax soap.

8. Continue stirring the soap mixture until it traces. At trace, if you pull the immersion blender out of the mixture and let it drip on the surface of the pot, the mixture will support the drip instead of allowing it to immediately settle back into the vat. Once trace occurs, add the essential oils. Continue stirring until the soap thickens like lemon curd or chilled pudding.

9. Pour the soap into the mold. Smooth the surface of the soap in the mold.

10. Cover the top of the mold with a silicone mat to hold in the heat. Cover all of this with a towel. Set the soap aside to complete the saponification process. The soap will go through a gel phase where the temperature of the soap rises, making the soap translucent. Then, as the saponification finishes, the soap will become opaque and firm. During this process, protect the surface underneath the mold from excessive heat. Smaller molds may not heat enough to go through a complete gel phase. The soap will be fine, though.

11. After 24 to 48 hours, the soap should be completely opaque with no translucent areas. The soap can be removed from the mold(s). The saponification process is almost done. It will continue inside the finished bars of soap for up to three weeks after the soap is made. If using a single loaf mold, wear gloves to cut the soap into 12 4-ounce bars. Stack the bars on a nonreactive tray to dry. Set aside for three weeks.

12. After three weeks, package the soap. It is now ready to use. However, after six months or more this bar will lather even better than when it was first made.

TO USE

Wet a shaving brush to create lather on the surface of the soap. Apply to the area being shaved.

Hairstyling Pomade

Beeswax shields your hair from the elements, protecting against moisture loss while aiding your self-expression. Whether your style is trim and conservative or flashy and creative, beeswax can help you express your unique style.

Hair pomade offers natural hold without the use of chemicals. It is a must for men's hairstyles that rely on lift and volume. Hair pomade tames the frizz while adding shine.

DILL
TIA

xxxxxxxx7800

1/14/2020

Item: 0010089501778 ((book)

Medium-Hold Pomade

YIELD: 3 (2-ounce) tins

INGREDIENTS

2 tablespoons beeswax

3 tablespoons kokum butter

2 tablespoons jojoba oil

1 tablespoon argan oil

20 drops sandalwood essential oil

20 drops rosemary essential oil

DIRECTIONS

1. Make a double boiler using a glass measuring cup. Simmer the beeswax, kokum butter, jojoba oil, and argan oil in the measuring cup over low heat, stirring until the beeswax is melted and the oils and butters combine. Remove the glass measuring cup from the saucepan. Add the essential oils.

2. Using a stick blender, blend the mixture as it cools so that it lightens in color and stiffens. Spoon the mixture into three 2-ounce tins. Allow this to cool completely. Label and date. The shelf life is 1 year.

TO USE

Scoop a pea-size amount into your hands and allow the pomade to melt at body temperature. Using your fingers, rub the pomade through your hair and style as usual.

Heavy-Hold Pomade

YIELD: 3 (2-ounce) tins

INGREDIENTS

3 tablespoons beeswax

2 tablespoons kokum butter

2 tablespoons jojoba oil

1 tablespoon argan oil

20 drops lime essential oil

20 drops rosemary essential oil

DIRECTIONS

1. Make a double boiler using a glass measuring cup. Place beeswax, kokum butter, jojoba oil, and argan oil in the cup. Simmer and stir over low heat until the beeswax is melted and the oils and butters combine. Remove the glass measuring cup from the saucepan. Add the essential oils.

2. Using a stick blender, blend the mixture as it cools so that it lightens in color and stiffens. Spoon the mixture into three 2-ounce tins. Allow this to cool completely. Label and date. This will last a year at room temperature.

TO USE

Scoop a pea-size amount into your hands and allow the pomade to melt at body temperature. Using your fingers, rub the pomade through your hair and style as usual.

✻ Moustache Wax

Moustache wax is pomade formulated especially for taming and conditioning the moustache. It's a must for handlebar moustaches but helps even regular moustaches stay manageable and tidy. It can minimize the formation of ice crystals on the moustache in winter weather.

The wax can be made softer by substituting 1 tablespoon of kokum butter for 1 tablespoon of beeswax or replacing 1 tablespoon of kokum butter with 1 tablespoon of avocado butter, which is a softer butter. It can be made firmer by adding 1 more tablespoon of beeswax in place of 1 of the tablespoon of kokum butter.

The pine resin offers superior hold, which is a must for handlebar moustache wax.

YIELD: 1 (4-ounce) tin

INGREDIENTS

2 tablespoons beeswax

2 tablespoons lanolin

2 tablespoons kokum butter

1 tablespoon pine resin

1 tablespoon argan oil

¼ teaspoon vitamin E oil

¼ teaspoon frankincense essential oil

¼ teaspoon cedar wood essential oil

DIRECTIONS

1. Make a double boiler using a glass measuring cup. Place the beeswax, lanolin, and kokum butter in the cup. In a second glass measuring cup, place the pine resin and argan oil, and place in the same saucepan. Simmer the saucepan on low heat until the pine resin and beeswax have both melted.

2. Turn off the saucepan and remove the glass measuring cups. Add the pine resin–argan oil mixture to the beeswax mixture, stirring constantly. Add the vitamin E and essential oils. Continue stirring until the mixture becomes thick and pale, like toffee.

3. Spoon into a 4-ounce tin. Label and date. This will last a year at room temperature.

TO USE

Melt a pea-size amount between your fingers and spread in your moustache, shaping as you apply the moustache wax.

❋ Beard Balm

Beard balm is a leave-in conditioner that softens, moisturizes, and helps style your beard. The beeswax in beard balm offers a light to medium hold, but its main job is to seal in moisture. A well-made beard balm will also condition the skin, leaving it soft and moisturized. Beard balm is a thicker, more moisturizing product than beard oil.

This beard balm contains vetiver, a strong, smoky-scented essential oil that is beneficial for skin care. The balm is woodsy, with a hint of smoke and lime.

YIELD: 1 (4-ounce) tin

INGREDIENTS

2 tablespoons beeswax

1 tablespoon shea butter

1 tablespoon cocoa butter

2 tablespoons avocado butter

2 tablespoons mango butter

2 tablespoons argan oil

10 drops sandalwood essential oil

30 drops lime essential oil

20 drops frankincense essential oil

2 drops of vetiver essential oil

DIRECTIONS

1. Make a double boiler using a glass measuring cup. Simmer the beeswax, the butters, and the argan oil in the cup over low heat until the beeswax and butters melt. Stir together to fully incorporate the beeswax with the butters and oil. Remove from heat.

2. Stir the mixture as it cools to just warm to prevent it from becoming too hard. While it is still warm, add the essential oils. Mix well.

3. Spoon the completed beard balm into a 4-ounce tin. Label and date the tin. Allow the beard balm to firm before using. The beard balm will last a year at room temperature.

TO USE

To apply, scrape a dime-size amount of the beard balm out of the tin with your finger nail. Rub the beard balm between your fingers to soften it. Rub your fingers through your beard to distribute the beard balm evenly. Use a comb to redistribute throughout and to style your beard.

Chapter 5

BEESWAX IN THE APOTHECARY

*Just as bees make honey from thyme, the
strongest and driest of herbs, so do the wise profit
from the most difficult of experiences.*

—Plato

Beeswax goes hand in hand with health and wellness. It's:

* Moisturizing

* A humectant

* Antimicrobial

* Anti-inflammatory

* Non-comedogenic

* Analgesic

Beeswax is naturally moisturizing and protecting. Just as it protects wood and leather from the harmful effects of the environment, it also protects our skin by sealing in moisture to protect against dehydration and the harmful effects of the external environment.

Beeswax is naturally antimicrobial. It has been used medicinally for thousands of years. Beeswax was used in the embalming process to prevent decay, deterring both moisture and bacteria. The Egyptian Coptic word for wax, "*mum,*" is thought by some to be where we get the English word, "mummy," so central was beeswax to the embalming process.

Beeswax offers texture and stability to herb-infused oils and medicinal preparations. The propolis and honey residues left in unfiltered, golden beeswax increases the soothing, antimicrobial, and moisturizing benefits.

Beeswax also acts as a binding and thickening agent, holding ingredients together so that they can be applied as an ointment or a salve to the skin. Beeswax has been listed in the official *Pharmacopeia*, the pharmacists' recipe book, for centuries.

Beeswax also has strong analgesic and anti-inflammatory actions, making it a popular ingredient in topical medicines for pain and inflammation. Yellow beeswax contains large amounts of vitamin A, an important vitamin that helps our skin manufacture collagen.

Scientific studies have found beeswax to be beneficial in treating diaper rash burns, rashes, psoriasis, and other skin conditions.

Medicinal Plants

Herbal remedies are plant-based medicines. Beeswax contains some natural, plant based-benefits derived from the bees' use of medicinal plants. However, when making remedies for the home apothecary, specific plants are utilized for precise, beneficial actions. Beeswax is an adjunct ingredient that contributes to texture and absorption.

Many of the healing components in plants are soluble in oil. Just as in making cosmetics, by infusing dried plant material in oil, we can extract these oil-soluble, restorative compounds. The usual ratio is 1 part dried plant material to 2 parts oil. It's important to use dried plant material when making infused oil. See page 62 for how to make herb-infused oil.

Up until now, the infused oils used in the recipes in this book have been single herbs infused in the oil. However, when making medicinal preparations, often more than one herb is used in each formulation since the herbs work in synergy. Each herb enhances the action of the other herbs used in the formula. When a recipe calls for more than one herb, there are two ways you can infuse the oils with the herbs.

The first way is to infuse oils with single herbs, making a "simple" infusion. This is the way most herbalists infuse oils. By making simple infusions, the infused oils become ingredients for future recipes. There are an infinite number of combinations that can be made with a few simple infusions.

Alternatively, you can infuse the combined herbs in the oil for each recipe, making just enough for that recipe. While the recipes may call for different carrier oils in this section of the book, virgin olive oil, sweet almond oil, or sunflower oil can be used interchangeably. See Chapter 10 on page 258 for the specific qualities that each oil and herb brings to the recipe so that you can make informed substitutions.

Herbal Ointments

An ointment is a mixture of wax and oil with herbs and sometimes essential oils. The texture of an ointment is semi-solid but somewhat softer than a balm or a salve, allowing it to be easily spread on a wound or a sore without causing pain. Herbal ointments melt at body temperature.

✳ Diaper Rash Ointment

Commercial diaper creams contain petrolatum, a petroleum-based gel—not exactly the nontoxic salve you want for your baby's tender skin. On the other hand, beeswax is nontoxic. It allows the skin to breathe, as it provides a vapor barrier to protect baby's hinder parts.

Calendula is skin healing, analgesic, and anti-inflammatory, making it soothing yet gentle for babies.

YIELD: 2 (2-ounce) tins

INGREDIENTS

2 tablespoons beeswax

4 tablespoons calendula-infused olive oil

2 tablespoons dandelion-infused olive oil

2 tablespoons cocoa butter

¾ teaspoon non-nano zinc oxide powder

10 drops frankincense essential oil

6 drops lavender essential oil

½ teaspoon vitamin E oil

DIRECTIONS

1. Make a double boiler using a glass measuring cup. Simmer the beeswax, infused oils, and cocoa butter in the cup until the beeswax and cocoa butter melt. Stir the ingredients together until well blended.

2. Add the zinc oxide powder. Using a stick blender, blend the zinc oxide powder into the oils and beeswax until they are well blended.

3. Remove from the heat and stir in the essential oils and the vitamin E oil.

4. Transfer the blended ingredients to two 2-ounce tins. Using two smaller containers rather than one larger container minimizes contamination of the tin with use. Label and date. The diaper rash ointment will last year if unopened. If the diaper rash ointment smells "off," discard and make a fresh batch.

TO USE

Apply on clean, dry skin before diapering.

🌾 Boo Boo Antimicrobial Ointment

The herbs in this antimicrobial ointment are styptic, helping to stop bleeding and minimize bruising. They promote rapid healing of minor cuts and scrapes and minimize infection. Since this has no chemical antibiotics, its use doesn't increase antibiotic resistance. For more serious injuries, consult your medical professional.

YIELD: 1 (4-ounce) jar

INGREDIENTS

1 tablespoon comfrey-infused oil

2 tablespoons calendula-infused oil

1 tablespoon plantain-infused oil

2 tablespoons yarrow-infused oil

2 tablespoons shea butter

2 tablespoons beeswax

¼ teaspoon vitamin E oil

10 drops tea tree essential oil

10 drops lavender essential oil

10 drops peppermint essential oil

DIRECTIONS

1. Make a double boiler using a glass measuring cup. Simmer the infused oils, shea butter, and beeswax in the glass measuring cup over low heat to melt the shea butter and beeswax. Remove from the heat. Stir the mixture while it cools to prevent the beeswax from clumping.

2. When the mixture is just warm to the touch, stir in the vitamin E and essential oils. Pour this mixture into a 4-ounce jar or a tin with a tight-fitting lid. Label and date. This will last for a year at room temperature.

TO USE

Wash the wound with soap and water. Dry well. Apply this ointment in a thin layer. Cover to keep the area clean and dry. Use this for minor cuts, scrapes, or bruises. For serious wounds, please consult your medical professional.

🦟 Calamine Ointment

Calamine lotion is the old standby remedy for itchy skin, bug bites, chicken pox, and poison ivy. It is soothing and cooling to the skin, relieving the burning and inflammation that accompanies these maladies. The active ingredient in calamine lotion is zinc oxide, with a pinch of iron oxide to give it the traditional pink color. You can make it at home.

While calamine lotion, a water-based preparation, can be made fresh as needed, this calamine ointment is shelf stable and can be made ahead and kept on hand for emergencies.

YIELD: 1 (4-ounce) or 2 (2-ounce) tins

INGREDIENTS

1 tablespoon shea butter

3 tablespoons sunflower oil

1 teaspoon dried calendula petals

1 teaspoon dried, crumbled plantain leaf

1 teaspoon dried rose petals

1 tablespoon beeswax

¼ teaspoon vitamin E oil

1 tablespoon zinc oxide

2 teaspoons pink kaolin clay

DIRECTIONS

1. Make a double boiler using a glass measuring cup. Simmer the shea butter and sunflower oil in the measuring cup over low heat, melting the shea butter and sunflower oil together. Stir in the

dried petals and plantain leaf. Simmer the water in the saucepan for about one hour to infuse the oil with the herbs. Allow this to cool naturally, until just warm. Strain the herbs from the oil, returning the oil to the glass measuring cup.

2. Return the measuring cup to the saucepan and simmer to warm the oils. Add the beeswax to the oils and stir to melt the beeswax completely. Add the vitamin E and stir to combine.

3. Stir the zinc oxide and the clay into the beeswax mixture. Use a stick blender or whisk to remove any lumps of powdered clay or zinc.

4. Once the mixture is smooth, pour into a tin(s). Label and date. This will last a year at room temperature.

TO USE

Apply as a soothing salve to itchy skin, bites, and rashes. If exposed to poison ivy, wash the skin first with soap and water and pat dry before applying.

🦟 Bug Bite Relief Stick

Allowing older children to control their own mosquito bite relief helps them feel less fussy and fearful when mosquitoes, chiggers, and other biting insects are around. Use push-up containers for this recipe to keep the top of the stick sanitary and prevent microbial contamination. Smaller amounts mean that if the stick is compromised, all the medicine isn't wasted.

YIELD: 2 (2-ounce) push-up container plus 1 (½-ounce) tin

INGREDIENTS

1 tablespoon dried, crushed plantain leaves

1 tablespoon dried, crumbled rose petals

1 tablespoon dried, crumbled dandelion flowers

3 tablespoons hemp seed oil

1 tablespoon shea butter

1 tablespoon beeswax

¼ teaspoon vitamin E oil

20 drops peppermint essential oil

DIRECTIONS

1. Make a double boiler using a glass measuring cup. Simmer the plantain leaves, rose petals, dandelion flowers, and hemp seed oil in the cup on low heat for one hour to infuse the oil with the herbs. Allow the herbs and oil to cool naturally. Strain the herbs out of the oil, reserving the oil. Compost the herbs.

2. Heat the oil in the glass cup double boiler on low heat. Add the shea butter and beeswax to the infused oil. Allow the beeswax to melt fully. Add the vitamin E. Remove from the heat. Allow to cool slightly. Add the peppermint essential oil.

3. Pour into two 1-ounce push-up containers, plus a ½-ounce tin for your purse. Label and date. This will last for a year at room temperature.

Note: For children under five, reduce the essential oil to 5 drops.

TO USE

Rub on insect bites and stings as often as necessary to reduce inflammation and swelling, and remove the itch.

🦟 Nick Stick Styptic

A styptic is applied to the skin to stop bleeding. Commercial styptic pencils are made from alum, an aluminum salt. For those avoiding aluminum, this styptic stick will soothe the nicks, prevent razor burn, and staunch bleeding quickly. Its special ingredient is yarrow *(Achillea millefolium)*, often called "wound wort" and "soldier's wort" because of its unique ability to stop bleeding fast. Yarrow is also antiseptic, antimicrobial, and encourages the skin to repair itself.

INGREDIENTS

2 tablespoons dried yarrow flowers and leaves

1 tablespoon dried calendula flowers

3 tablespoons sunflower oil

1 tablespoon shea butter

1 tablespoon beeswax

½ teaspoon vitamin E oil

12 drops frankincense essential oil

DIRECTIONS

1. Make a double boiler using a glass measuring cup. Simmer the yarrow and calendula flowers with the sunflower oil in the cup over low heat for one hour to infuse the oil with the herbs. Allow the herbs and oil to cool naturally. Strain the herbs out of the oil, reserving the oil. Compost the herbs.

2. Return the glass cup to the saucepan of water. Simmer the infused oil, shea butter, and beeswax in the cup over low heat. Melt the beeswax with the oil and stir to combine. Add the vitamin E. Remove from the heat. Allow to cool slightly. Add the frankincense essential oil.

3. Pour into 2 1-ounce push-up containers. Label and date. This will last a year at room temperature.

TO USE

Splash affected area with cold water and pat dry. Apply a small dap of the nick stick to any nicks or scratches to staunch bleeding.

🐝 Cold Relief Chest Rub

Decongestant chest rubs are a part of childhood cold relief. They loosen chest congestion while clearing sinuses with their aromatic oils. However, these products are no longer recommended for children due to concerns over the effects of the strong menthol vapors on children's breathing.

You can make a gentler version using infused oils in the place of the menthol crystals common in the over-the-counter product.

YIELD: 1 (2-ounce) tin

INGREDIENTS

1 tablespoon crushed eucalyptus leaves

1 tablespoon crushed peppermint leaves

1 teaspoon rosemary leaves

1 teaspoon thyme leaves

4 tablespoons jojoba oil

1 tablespoon beeswax

¼ teaspoon vitamin E oil

10 drops eucalyptus radiata essential oil

3 drops peppermint essential oil

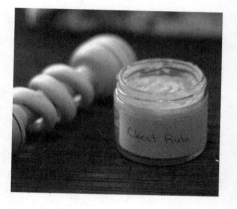

DIRECTIONS

1. Make a double boiler using a glass measuring cup. Simmer the eucalyptus, peppermint, rosemary, and thyme leaves in jojoba oil in the cup for one hour. Turn off the heat. Allow the mixture to cool naturally. Strain the herbs out of the oil. Return the oil to the glass measuring cup, in the saucepan, and gently heat the oil.

2. Add the beeswax and stir the oil until the beeswax is melted. Stir in the vitamin E and essential oils.

3. Mix thoroughly. Pour into a 2-ounce tin. Label and date. This will last a year at room temperature.

4. Omit the essential oils for children under 5. Essential oils may be added for older children and for adults.

Rub on the chest and upper back to relieve sinus congestion and chest congestion when there are cold symptoms. If the congestion persists or there is difficulty breathing, consult a medical professional.

Cayenne-Pine Ointment

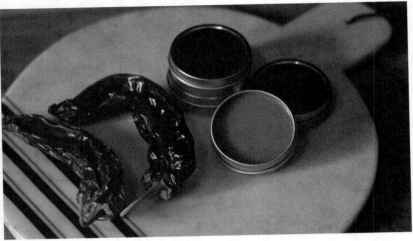

For arthritic pain, swollen joints, muscle strains, gouty swelling, or painful muscles, this ointment will bring warmth to the area, increase circulation, and help relieve inflammation and pain.

YIELD: 1 (4-ounce) tin

INGREDIENTS

6 tablespoons olive oil

1 teaspoon cayenne pepper powder

1 tablespoon ginger powder

2 tablespoons beeswax

1 tablespoon pine resin

¼ teaspoon vitamin E oil

10 drops spruce bud essential oil

10 drops rosemary essential oil

1. Make a double boiler using a glass measuring cup. Place the olive oil in the cup, in the saucepan, on low heat. Add the powdered spices. Infuse the olive oil with the powdered cayenne pepper and ginger for one hour. After one hour, turn off the heat. Allow the oil to cool to just warm. Strain the powdered herbs through a cloth and reserve the oil.

2. Return the oil to the glass cup. Warm the oil slightly in the double boiler. Add the beeswax and pine resin. Continue heating gently just until the pine resin and beeswax melt fully. Stir together.

3. Add the vitamin E. Remove from heat and stir gently while the mixture cools. While it is still soft and warm to the touch, stir in the essential oils.

4. Spoon this into a 4-ounce tin. Label and date. This will last one year at room temperature.

TO USE

Apply to painful, swollen joints, aches, and muscles. Rub into the skin.

Do not use on broken skin. It can cause stinging. Wash hands after using. Avoid touching eyes after use. It can cause a burning sensation on mucous membranes. On unbroken skin, it will increase circulation. With regular use it can reduce swelling and inflammation.

Herbal Salves

Salves combine herbs with oils and wax to make a semi-solid product. Salves have a firmer texture than ointments, but are not as firm as balms. Salves melt at body temperature, allowing the active constituents of the herbs to be absorbed through the skin. The oil and wax both have moisturizing and protective benefits. Combined with herbs that have medicinal actions, their benefits increase.

Herbal salves are generally 25 percent beeswax.

🌠 Gardener's Salve

Gardeners and others who work with their hands end up with nicks and cuts, slivers, and abrasions that seem to take a long time to heal. The injury is compounded because during gardening season, there is no break in the abuse. Weeding, planting, and mulching all take their toll. This salve, applied at night, can help to moisturize and heal those hardworking hands.

YIELD: 1 (4-ounce) tin

INGREDIENTS

2 tablespoons hemp seed oil

1 tablespoon mango butter

1 teaspoon dried chamomile flowers

1 tablespoon fresh St. John's wort flowers

1 teaspoon dried yarrow flowers

1 tablespoon beeswax

¼ teaspoon vitamin E oil

1 tablespoon rose hip seed oil

25 drops marjoram essential oil

10 drops tea tree essential oil

10 drops frankincense essential oil

DIRECTIONS

1. Make a double boiler using a glass measuring cup. Simmer the hemp seed oil, mango butter, and herbs in the cup for one hour to melt the mango butter and infuse the herbs into the oil. Stir the herbs to moisten completely. Remove from the heat.

2. Allow the contents of the measuring cup to reduce in temperature so that you can handle the cup without being burned. Strain the herbs from the oils and discard, reserving the oil.

3. Return the oil to the measuring cup and the measuring cup to the saucepan. Add the beeswax. Simmer the saucepan just

until the beeswax melts. Remove from the heat. Allow to cool slightly, stirring to prevent the beeswax from clumping together.

4. Add the vitamin E, rose hip seed oil, and essential oils. Mix well.

5. Pour this into a 4-ounce tin. Label and date. This will last a year at room temperature.

TO USE

Apply salve to clean hands as often as needed.

Black Drawing Salve

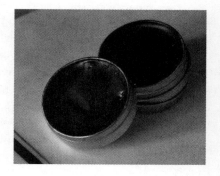

Drawing salve helps the body to push foreign objects out by counter irritation, which increases circulation to the area. Drawing salve can also be used on spider bites and boils to draw the inflammation to the surface of the skin, where it can be cleaned out.

In this recipe, plantain and pine resin increase circulation and help draw slivers to the surface of the skin, while calendula promotes good drainage of the wound and helps the body to heal the surrounding tissue.

YIELD: 2 (2-ounce) tins

INGREDIENTS

3 tablespoons olive oil

1 tablespoon shea butter

1 teaspoon dried calendula blossoms

1 teaspoon dried, crushed plantain leaves

1 tablespoon beeswax

1 tablespoon pine resin

1 tablespoon pink kaolin clay

1 tablespoon activated charcoal

¼ teaspoon vitamin E oil

25 drops frankincense essential oil

DIRECTIONS

1. Make a double boiler using a glass measuring cup. Simmer the olive oil, shea butter, and herbs in the cup for one hour to melt the shea butter and infuse the herbs into the oil. Stir the herbs to moisten completely. Remove from the heat.

2. Allow the contents of the measuring cup to reduce in temperature so that you can handle the cup without being burned. Strain the herbs from the oils and discard, reserving the oil.

3. Return the oil to the measuring cup and the measuring cup to the saucepan. Add the beeswax and the pine resin. Simmer the saucepan just until the beeswax and pine resin melt together. Stir to blend well. Remove from the heat.

4. Stir in the clay and the charcoal. Stir gently, as the charcoal has a tendency to become airborne. Stir until the powders are completely mixed and there are no lumps.

5. Add the vitamin E and frankincense essential oil. Mix well.

6. Pour this into tins. Label and date. This will last one year at room temperature.

TO USE

Apply the salve to clean, dry skin. Cover with a bandage. Reapply every four hours until the foreign object is removed. If infection or redness increases, consult with your medical professional.

🦟 Bug-Be-Gone Insect Repellent

Bug repellent is generally water based and needs to be reapplied after strenuous activity or water sports. This beeswax formula is water resistant and will be effective against biting insects longer than water-based preparations.

YIELD: 2 (2-ounce) tins

INGREDIENTS

4 tablespoons olive oil

2 tablespoons mango butter

¼ cup finely chopped fresh mint leaves

¼ cup finely chopped fresh lemon balm leaves

2 tablespoons beeswax

¼ teaspoon vitamin E oil

25 drops tea tree essential oil

20 drops lemon verbena essential oil

15 drops lavender essential oil

DIRECTIONS

1. Place olive oil and mango butter in a glass measuring cup. Add the herbs and stir to moisten completely. Place the measuring cup into a small saucepan with water and simmer for one hour to infuse the herbs in the oil and melt the mango butter. Remove from the heat. Allow the contents of the measuring cup to reduce in temperature so that you can handle the cup without being burned. Strain the herbs from the oils and discard, reserving the oil.

2. Return the oil to the measuring cup and the measuring cup the saucepan. Add the beeswax. Simmer the saucepan just until the beeswax melts. Remove from the heat.

3. Add the vitamin E and essential oils. Mix well.

4. Pour this into tins. Label and date. This will last for one year at room temperature.

Note: If using this preparation with babies and children under five, omit the essential oils.

TO USE

Apply to bare skin, especially the back of the neck and the back of hands and ankles to discourage mosquitoes from biting.

✳ Calendula-Chamomile Sunburn Salve

Calendula and chamomile are soothing to minor burns. This salve reduces moisture loss while improving the body's ability to regenerate the skin tissue after sunburn.

YIELD: 2 (4-ounce) tins

INGREDIENTS

½ cup olive oil

2 tablespoons avocado butter

2 tablespoons dried calendula blossoms

2 tablespoons dried chamomile blossoms

2 tablespoons beeswax

¼ teaspoon vitamin E oil

10 drops lavender essential oil

5 drops rosemary essential oil

DIRECTIONS

1. Make a double boiler using a glass measuring cup. Place the olive oil and avocado butter in the cup. Add the herbs to the olive oil mixture and stir to moisten the herbs completely. Place the measuring cup into a small saucepan with water in it. Simmer the water in the saucepan for one hour to melt the avocado butter and infuse the herbs into the oil. Remove from the heat. Allow the contents of the measuring cup to reduce in temperature so

that you can handle the cup without being burned. Strain the herbs from the oils and discard, reserving the oil.

2. Return the oil to the measuring cup and the measuring cup the saucepan. Add the beeswax. Simmer the saucepan just until the beeswax melts. Remove from the heat. Allow the mixture to cool while stirring to prevent the beeswax from clumping while it cools.

3. While the mixture is still warm to the touch, add the vitamin E and essential oils. Mix well.

4. Pour this into tins. Label and date. This will last for a year at room temperature.

TO USE

Cool the sunburn with cold cloths that have been soaked in water and wrung out. Continue applying cold compresses until much of the heat is gone from the sunburn. Once the sunburn has cooled, apply this salve to moisturize the skin and reduce any inflammation and pain. It will help the skin heal more quickly and reduce peeling.

DIY Skin Nourishing Sunscreen

This recipe for DIY sunscreen takes advantage of the natural SPF values and antioxidant qualities of natural oils, beeswax, and vegetable butters. Lavender, calendula, raspberry seed oil, and vitamin E are high in antioxidants to repair free radical damage. The addition of zinc oxide is optional. Add it to 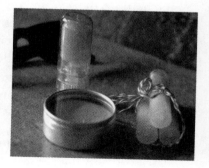 the recipe after the oils are mixed if you are spending a long time in the sun or if you need a broad spectrum sunscreen to protect from both UVA and UVB damage. Without the addition of zinc oxide, this sunscreen recipe has a natural SPF of about 15 and offers protection from UVB radiation only. With it, this recipe offers an SPF of 20 to 30.

YIELD: 1 (4-ounce) jar or tin

INGREDIENTS

2 tablespoons virgin olive oil

2 tablespoons hemp seed oil

2 tablespoons shea butter

2 tablespoons dried calendula blossoms

2 tablespoons beeswax

1 tablespoon raspberry seed oil

1 teaspoon vitamin E oil

25 drops lavender essential oil

1 tablespoon non–nano zinc oxide (optional) to increase the SPF to 20 (or use 1½ tablespoons to increase SPF to 30)

DIRECTIONS

1. Make a double boiler using a heat–proof glass measuring cup. Place olive oil, hemp seed oil, and shea butter in the cup. Crumble the calendula flowers and add them to the cup. Stir the herbs to moisten them completely. Place the measuring cup into a small saucepan with water in it. Simmer the water for one hour to melt the shea butter and infuse the herbs into the oils. Remove from the heat. Allow the contents of the measuring cup to reduce in temperature so that you can handle the cup without being burned. Strain the herbs from the oils and discard, reserving the oil.

2. Return the oil to the measuring cup and the measuring cup the saucepan. Add the beeswax. Simmer the saucepan just until the beeswax melts. Stir the infused oils so that the beeswax combines with the oils. Remove from the heat.

3. Allow the mixture to cool slightly. Stir it to prevent the beeswax from clumping together with the oils. While it is still warm to

the touch, stir in the raspberry seed oil, vitamin E , and essential oils. Stir to combine. Remove from the heat.

4. If using, stir zinc oxide powder into the oils with a spoon. Once the zinc oxide powder is moistened, use a stick blender to combine fully. Use a dust mask and gloves to protect from zinc oxide inhalation.

5. Pour the sunscreen mixture into a 4-ounce glass jar or tin. Label and date. This will last a year at room temperature.

TO USE

This sunscreen is oil based. It will feel a bit greasy going on but will quickly be absorbed by your skin. It is moisturizing. The zinc oxide blends in and won't leave a white paste on the surface of your skin. It is water resistant but may need to be reapplied with long sun exposure or after heavy sweating.

Herbal Lotions

Lotions are emulsified mixtures of oil and water. If you made Galen's Cold Cream (page 99), you've already had some experience making an herbal lotion. The following herbal lotions follow the same principles.

🌿 Magnesium Lotion

Magnesium is essential to cell functions. Your heart depends on it. Muscle aches, growing pains, and calf cramps can all be helped with magnesium supplementation. However, the best way to absorb magnesium into the body is through the skin, rather than through the intestines. Epsom salt baths are one way to get the benefits of magnesium. Putting magnesium lotion right where the ache or cramp is can offer quick relief.

Use this lotion after strenuous exercise to prevent muscle aches.

YIELD: 1 (8-ounce) glass jar

INGREDIENTS

Water phase

½ cup magnesium chloride flakes

1 teaspoon borax

3 tablespoons boiling water

Oil Phase

¼ cup coconut oil

1 tablespoon sunflower lecithin

2 tablespoons beeswax

3 tablespoons cocoa butter

DIRECTIONS

1. Add the magnesium flakes and borax to a glass measuring cup. Pour the boiling water into the magnesium-borax mixture and stir until it dissolves. It takes quite a bit of stirring to get the magnesium flakes to dissolve. This will create a thick liquid. Set aside to cool.

2. Make a double boiler using a 4-cup glass measuring cup. In the cup, combine the coconut oil, sunflower lecithin, beeswax, and cocoa butter and turn the heat to medium.

3. When the beeswax and cocoa butter are melted, remove the cup from the pan and let the mixture cool to room temperature. It should be slightly opaque. Stir it while it cools to prevent clumping. Using an immersion blender, start blending the oil mixture.

4. Slowly trickle the magnesium mixture into the vortex of the whirling oil mixture while blending constantly, until all the magnesium mixture is blended into the oil mixture and the lotion is thick and fluffy. Continue blending for 5 minutes. The mixture will become thick and opaque.

5. Place in the fridge to cool completely. Re-blend with the immersion blender if necessary to get a complete emulsion. Transfer to a glass jar for storage. Label and date.

6. This has no antimicrobial additives. It will keep in the fridge for about 2 months or at room temperature for a month.

TO USE

Apply to the skin after exercising, after a shower, or before bed.

🪰 Anti-Acne Lotion

Beeswax, honey, and propolis lotions are known to be healing to the skin, contributing to clear complexion. But oil-based salves are a little too heavy for skin troubled with acne. Try this light lotion with willow bark and calendula. Willow bark is astringent, antimicrobial, and anti-inflammatory, while calendula helps fluids move and encourages healthy skin.

YIELD: 1 (4-ounce) jar

INGREDIENTS

1 tablespoon crumbled dried calendula blossoms

1 tablespoon powdered dried willow bark

¼ cup vodka

¼ teaspoon borax

2 teaspoons beeswax

1 teaspoon raw honey

¼ teaspoon lanolin

2 tablespoons mango butter

1 tablespoons rose hip seed oil

1 teaspoon sea buckthorn oil

½ teaspoon vitamin E oil

10 drops lavender essential oil

10 drops frankincense essential oil

DIRECTIONS

1. In a half-cup mason jar, place the calendula blossoms, willow bark, and vodka. Cap tightly and set aside for two weeks, shaking daily. Strain the vodka from the herbs. Discard the herbs and retain the vodka.

2. Stir the borax into the infused vodka in a glass measuring cup. Warm the mixture to 90°F by placing the cup in a pan of hot tap water. Set aside.

3. In a second glass measuring cup, create a double boiler. Combine the beeswax, honey, lanolin, and mango butter in the cup. Heat the oils just enough to melt the beeswax and mango butter. Allow the oils to cool to 110°F. Stir the mixture while it cools. When it is no longer steaming and you can hold your hand against the side of the cup without burning your hand, add the rose hip seed oil, sea buckthorn oil, vitamin E, and essential oils. Stir well. The mixture will thicken as it cools.

4. When the mixture has cooled to 100°F, place an immersion blender in the cup and turn it on at its highest speed. In a slow, thin drizzle, pour the vodka–borax mixture into the vortex of the whirling oil mixture.

5. When most of the vodka has been added to the mixture and the cream looks thick and white, turn off the immersion blender.

6. Spoon the mixture into glass jars. The cream will thicken as it sets. Label and date.

7. This lotion has no preservatives. It should be kept in the fridge when not in use. It should last about a month. Discard if it shows signs of mold or begins to smell "off."

TO USE

Apply a small dab and massage into blemished skin.

Chapter 6

BEESWAX HOME COMFORTS

The bee is more honored than other animals, not because she labors, but because she labors for others.

—St. John Chrysostom

Beeswax has a long history of use in the home. Beyond lighting, beeswax was a vital component in wood polishes, finishes, and cleaning products, offering protection, lubrication, and durability. It has uses in the kitchen, too. It was traditionally used in food preservation and cooking.

Beeswax is included for hardness, gloss, and elasticity. By combining beeswax in different proportions to other ingredients, the hardness or malleability of the product can be manipulated.

While homecare products using beeswax go back hundreds of years, it isn't as simple as just reproducing the olden day's recipe for today's uses. Beeswax hasn't changed in thousands of years; however, the other ingredients in the old recipes have changed. Some of the older recipes wouldn't be considered safe today, with carcinogenic additives like cadmium, lead, and petroleum distillates. Other recipes seem easy enough to replicate, but the toxic and flammable fumes require special venting hoods and safety equipment. You don't want those fumes in your home.

Traditional recipes using natural beeswax include industrial solvents like turpentine and boiled linseed oil. These additives are not the same products that were used hundreds of years ago in traditional recipes.

Formerly, turpentine was distilled from natural pine sap. It was a therapeutic product used in medicine, animal care, and wood care products. The distillation process left behind rosin or pine resin, two additional beneficial and therapeutic products. Today's turpentine has no connection to its roots in traditional medicine. It is a simulated product filled with petroleum distillates, chemical dryers, and paint thinners. Today, true gum turpentine can be obtained only from specialty suppliers. You won't find it at the local hardware store.

Drying and Non-Drying Oils for Wood Care

Whether an oil is drying, non-drying, or somewhere in between depends on the unsaturated fats in the oil. Drying oils have more unsaturated fats, which form double-carbon bonds. These double-carbon bonds (C=C) react with iodine and are measured by an iodine number. Those oils with iodine numbers 130 or higher are considered drying oils. Those with iodine numbers below 115 are non-drying oils. The in-between oils are considered semi-drying.

Drying oils form a polymer film as they dry, sealing the surface with a moisture barrier. The drying potential of one of the drying oils can be increased by heating the oil so that a film forms on the top of the oil. This should be done very carefully to avoid burning the oil. The difference between raw linseed oil and boiled linseed oil is this heating of the oil. In the commercial product, heavy metals, petroleum distillates, and dryers are added to speed the drying time.

Drying oils include flax seed or linseed oil, hemp seed oil, grape seed oil, walnut oil, sunflower oil, and tung oil. Semi-drying oils include canola oil, pecan oil, safflower oil, and sesame oil. Non-drying oils include jojoba oil, olive oil, coconut oil, almond oil, avocado oil, and tallow.

Natural linseed or flaxseed oil is a drying oil that forms a thin polymer film as it slowly dries on the surface of wood. By boiling linseed oil, its drying qualities can be enhanced. However, today's boiled linseed oil has heavy metals, chemicals, and dryers added to speed the drying process.

Chemical additives in home-cleaning and workshop products present a challenge to those who desire to create a nontoxic home environment. Open a can of commercial paste wax to care for your hardwood floors and you'll immediately understand. These products must be used in a well-ventilated space. They are not safe to use around young children or pets. The toxic fumes can last for days in your home.

The recipes here offer sustainable alternatives to commercial products that won't leave you wearing a gas mask. Each recipe is made with natural beeswax and a few basic ingredients that you'll reuse for other recipes in this book. If any of the ingredients are problematic for your family, check the substitution suggestions in Chapter 10 for alternatives.

Wood Care

Oils used for wood care are divided into three categories: drying oils, semi-drying oils, and non-drying oils. Drying oils dry upon exposure to oxygen, forming a smooth polymer film on the surface of the wood. Non-drying oils are absorbed by the wood through capillary action, but excess oil must be wiped off. Semi-drying oils are both absorbed into the wood and form a thin polymer film on the surface of the wood. Excess oil will not fully dry on the wood surface and must be wiped off. Linseed oil is a drying oil, while mineral oil is non-drying.

Waxes form a moisture barrier on the surface of the wood. When blended with oil, beeswax is drawn into the wood by capillary action, forming a soft finish. Traditional wood polishes, waxes, and finishes utilize these natural properties to clean, condition, seal, and prevent cracking or checking in wood with changes in humidity.

Many polishes and preservatives include resins as well. Resins form a thin film over the surface of wood to add shine, scratch resistance, and water resistance, protecting the wood. Resins are used on wood that gets hard use, like table tops, floors, drawer fronts, and cupboard fronts, to maintain their shine, resist scratching, and protect from water marks.

🐝 Paste Wax for Wooden Floors

Wooden floors are warm and comforting. This beeswax-based polish will protect them and help them resist scratching and moisture. Use twice a year to protect hardwood floors and keep them looking good.

Natural gum turpentine is a different product than the turpentine you get at the hardware store. It is the distilled volatile oils that are boiled off natural pine pitch, leaving behind pine resin. The volatile oils contain essential oil of pine and terpinene. It smells pleasant, like a pine forest on a summer afternoon. It is not toxic. Gum turpentine can be purchased from specialty foresters or art supply stores (see Resources on page 278). Do not substitute synthetic turpentine in this recipe.

On light-colored wood, use white, filtered beeswax in this recipe. Yellow beeswax will leave the wood with a yellow cast with repeat applications of wax. Yellow beeswax is suitable for darker, heavier wood.

YIELD: 3 (4-ounce) tins

INGREDIENTS

¾ cup beeswax

2 tablespoons carnauba wax

½ cup natural gum turpentine

DIRECTIONS

1. Make a double boiler using a tin can. Add the beeswax and carnauba wax to the can. Warm over medium heat to melt the wax together. When the mixture is fully melted, remove from the heat.

2. Slowly drizzle in the gum turpentine. Stir while it cools to prevent the beeswax from hardening into lumps.

3. Spoon into tins.

TO USE

Fully clean the floor with a damp mop. Allow the floor to air dry fully.

Apply paste wax with a damp cloth. Rub in the paste wax in the direction of the wood grain. Use a thin coat of wax and wipe off any residual wax on the floor surface. Leave for one hour to allow the wax to penetrate the floor surface.

Buff with a buffing cloth or use an electric floor polisher. This dries to a hard, scratch-resistant finish that resists wear.

On a finished floor, this should be applied twice annually. On a new floor, this should be applied once a week for a month, then once a month for a year, then twice a year thereafter.

Furniture Polish

This is a creamy polish to apply to fine furniture, dining room tables, coffee tables, cabinet doors, or chairs. Once it is fully dry and cured, it will not transfer any oil to people sitting on the chairs.

YIELD: 1 (8-ounce) jar

INGREDIENTS

3 tablespoons beeswax

1 tablespoon grated soap flakes

¼ cup very hot water

½ cup natural gum turpentine

2 tablespoons d-limonene

DIRECTIONS

1. Make a double boiler using a tin can. Add the beeswax to the can and melt over medium heat. In a separate can, melt soap flakes in the hot water. Remove the beeswax from the heat and slowly drizzle the gum turpentine into the beeswax. Continue stirring until there are no beeswax lumps. Slowly add the d-limonene to the beeswax mixture, stirring while you add it.

2. Slowly drizzle the soapy water mixture into the beeswax mixture, stirring constantly until well blended. The mixture will thicken, becoming creamy.

3. Pour into an 8-ounce, wide-mouth glass jar with a tight-fitting lid. Store in a cool place. Keep well covered. If the polish separates in storage, shake it well before using.

TO USE

Use a soft cotton cloth to apply and rub the furniture polish onto the wood surface. Use a toothbrush to get into small crevices and cover every wood surface. Rub in well, completely covering the wood. Allow this to dry for 30 minutes. Wipe off excess. Buff with a soft cloth to remove any residual polish and restore shine.

English Polish for Furniture

Wax finishes form a deep layer of wax that penetrates the pores of the wood. Beeswax finishes create a deep patina that you can see down into. Beeswax leaves a satin finish that is tough and impermeable to water and alcohol. However, it will be damaged by heat, so take care to use protective mats and coasters to insulate the surface from heat damage.

This is the very best polish to use on bare wood. It is nontoxic and food safe when made with pure gum turpentine.

YIELD: 1 (8-ounce) jar

INGREDIENTS

½ cup beeswax

½ cup gum turpentine

DIRECTIONS

1. Grate the beeswax into fine shreds or use beeswax pastilles. Place the beeswax in a glass pint jar with a tight-fitting lid. Pour the gum turpentine over the beeswax. Shake well. Allow a few days for the beeswax to dissolve in the gum turpentine.

2. Shake the mixture a few times a day to distribute the turpentine and beeswax. The mixture will form a liquid wax.

TO APPLY

Put a thin amount of liquid wax on very fine steel wool. Apply to the wood surface, rubbing with the grain, in a thin, even coat. Leave it to dry for one hour. Using a soft cotton cloth, buff the surface of the dried wax in a circular motion. If you are waxing new furniture or refinishing older wood, repeat the application of waxing, drying, and buffing several times, allowing 24 hours between coats. To maintain a wax finish, wax once a year or when the finish seems dull.

The general rule for applying deep wax finishes on new fine furniture is:

* Once a day for a week

* Once a week for a month

* Once a month for a year

* Once a year thereafter

Beeswax in the Kitchen

Beeswax is a nontoxic ingredient for kitchen maintenance, cleaning, food storage, and cooking. Combined with other healthful ingredients, beeswax can replace endocrine-disrupting plastics, chemical solvents, cleaners, and wood conditioners.

🐝 Wooden Spoon Cleaner and Conditioner

Make a nontoxic wood cleaner and conditioner for wooden spoons and utensils. Walnut oil was traditionally used as a wood finish in France. It is a drying oil and forms a protective polymer film on the surface of the wood as it dries. Those allergic to tree nuts can substitute grape seed oil for the walnut oil in this recipe. Grape seed oil has the same strong drying qualities as walnut oil. The orange essential oil has antimicrobial activity and lends its scent to the finished product.

YIELD: 1 (4-ounce) tin or jar

INGREDIENTS

3 tablespoons beeswax

1 tablespoon coconut oil

4 tablespoons walnut oil

¼ teaspoon vitamin E oil

30 drops sweet orange essential oil

DIRECTIONS

1. Make a double boiler using a glass measuring cup. Add the beeswax and coconut oil to the cup. Melt the beeswax and coconut oil together over medium heat. Drizzle the walnut oil into the beeswax, stirring constantly. If the beeswax solidifies, continue stirring until it melts again. Remove from the heat source.

2. Allow the mixture to cool slightly, then add the vitamin E and orange essential oil. Stir well to incorporate.

3. Pour into a 4-ounce jar or tin. Allow the wooden spoon cleaner and conditioner to solidify.

TO USE

Wipe on clean, dry wooden spoons and utensils. Allow the tools to sit for one hour or overnight. Then wipe off any excess polish with a soft cloth. Buff until the tools are no longer tacky. Weekly use will prevent the tools from drying out, cracking, or losing their strength.

🐝 Food-Safe Wooden Cutting Board Polish and Conditioner

Wooden cutting boards are naturally antimicrobial. They are a better choice than plastic for food preparation. But don't put them in the dishwasher. Instead, wash them in the sink with hot soapy water and dry immediately.

To maintain their strength, use this food–safe polish and conditioner once a month.

YIELD: 1 (4-ounce) tin or 2 (2-ounce) jars

INGREDIENTS

2 tablespoons beeswax

2 tablespoons jojoba oil

4 tablespoons coconut oil

¼ teaspoon lemon essential oil

DIRECTIONS

1. Make a double boiler using a glass cup. Add the beeswax, jojoba oil, and coconut oil to the cup. Melt together over medium heat. Remove from the heat as soon as the beeswax is fully melted. Stir this together well.

2. Add the lemon essential oil. Stir well.

3. Pour into a tin or jars.

TO USE

Apply the polish to clean, dry cutting boards. Allow this to sit on the surface of the board for one hour. Wipe off with a dry, lint-free cloth. Apply once a month.

Keeping Copper Clean

Decorative copper pieces may be lacquered by the manufacturer to prevent tarnishing. A lacquer finish prevents oxidization so lacquered copper will appear shiny with no discoloration over time. Decorative lacquered copper should never be polished or waxed. These pieces need special care so that the delicate lacquer finish is not damaged. They can be cleaned with mild soap and water followed by drying with a soft cloth.

Lacquered dishes used for food should have the lacquer removed before using. You can do this by boiling the piece in a stainless steel pot with water to which you've added 1 tablespoon of washing soda. Boil for 30 minutes. Remove the pieces from the hot water and allow them to cool. Wash in mild dish soap and dry thoroughly.

If your copper pieces darken or develop a green-blue patina, they can be cleaned using a paste of lemon juice, salt, and flour. In fact, all copper pieces should be cleaned of verdigris before applying a protective wax finish because verdigris is toxic. You can use the Pre-Treatment Copper-Cleaning Paste (below) to make your copper pieces food-safe. Note: Unlined copper pots should not remain in contact with food.

🦟 Pre-Treatment Copper-Cleaning Paste

YIELD: 1 pre-treatment

INGREDIENTS

Juice of one lemon

1 tablespoon extra-fine salt

1 to 2 tablespoons flour

Seal for Copper and Brass (page 165)

DIRECTIONS

1. This cleaner should be made fresh as needed. Do not try to store it. Combine ingredients in a small pottery bowl, adding just enough flour to make a thick but spreadable paste.

2. Using a soft cloth, apply a small amount of the tarnish cleaning paste to the copper surface. Work the tarnish remover into the surface by rubbing briskly with a cloth. Rinse the copper object. Dry with a towel.

3. Apply a thin coating of Seal for Copper and Brass to prevent oxidization and maintain the luster.

🐝 Seal for Copper and Brass

A thin seal of beeswax will maintain the shine on freshly cleaned copper or brass pieces while preventing oxidization. Pieces should be fully dry before applying the beeswax.

YIELD: 1 (2-ounce) jar

INGREDIENTS

3 tablespoons beeswax

4 tablespoons 99% rubbing alcohol

DIRECTIONS

1. Grate beeswax finely or use beeswax pastilles. Place in a pint-size glass jar. Add the rubbing alcohol. Cap tightly. Shake the jar every few hours until the beeswax fully dissolves in the rubbing alcohol.

2. Apply the liquid wax to the brass or copper in a thin layer, using a soft cloth. Allow it to dry. Buff to a hard shine.

3. Replace the wax covering as necessary. This wax can be kept for months without loss of quality. Shake well before using.

🐝 Granite Countertop Polish

Your granite countertops need the same kind of polishing and sealing as your wooden table. A wax finish will make them impervious to water and marking. The wax will fill in scratches and resist fingerprints. Most commercial granite polishes are acrylic and silicone-based and have added chemical dryers.

YIELD: 1 (4-ounce) tin

INGREDIENTS

3 tablespoons beeswax

1 tablespoon orange wax

2 tablespoons d-limonene

3 tablespoons hemp seed oil

DIRECTIONS

1. Make a double boiler with a glass measuring cup. Heat the beeswax and orange wax in the double boiler until just melted.

2. Slowly drizzle in the d-limonene. Slowly drizzle in the hemp seed oil. Stir until all the beeswax is melted and the mixture is completely liquid.

3. Pour into a 4-ounce tin. Allow the mixture to solidify before using.

4. This will last indefinitely if stored in a cool, dry place.

TO USE

Clean and dry your granite countertops or sinks. The granite surface must be completely dry before polishing. Using a soft cloth, apply a thin layer of polish in a circular motion over the entire surface. Allow it to dry for 30 minutes to an hour. When the granite surface is fully dry, buff with a clean cloth, using a circular motion. Remove all excess wax by dry buffing.

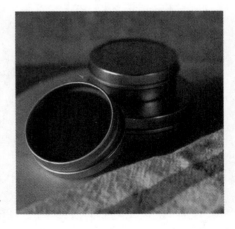

🐝 Beeswax Food Wrap

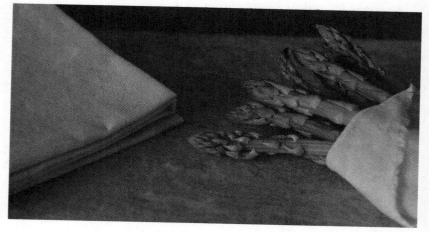

Forget the plastic bags and cling wrap. Using reusable, bees-wax-impregnated cloth, you can save money and avoid the use of endocrine-disrupting plastic.

This recipe makes four food wraps that are big enough to cover a bowl or wrap a sandwich with. Double the recipe when you make it and include enough cotton fabric to make beeswax food wraps for a friend, too.

The pine resin is what makes the cloth cling to a bowl. It's sticky but dissolves in oil. Use a little oil to help with clean up.

YIELD: 4 (14 x 14-inch) food wraps

INGREDIENTS

¼ cup beeswax

2 tablespoons pine resin

1 tablespoon jojoba oil

4 (14 x 14-inch) squares of 100% cotton muslin fabric

EQUIPMENT

Parchment paper

Baking sheet

1-inch-wide natural bristle, disposable paintbrush

Clothes drying rack

DIRECTIONS

1. Make a double boiler using a glass measuring cup. Melt the beeswax and pine resin together in the cup, over medium heat. When the beeswax and pine resin are liquid, drizzle the jojoba oil into the mixture while stirring. You may need to scrape the pine resin off the bottom of the jar and stir it into the beeswax once the mixture is melted. Leave the beeswax mixture in the double boiler and the heat turned on low to keep the mixture liquid while you work with the fabric pieces.

2. Wash the cotton muslin pieces well to remove the sizing and hang to dry. Press them with a steam iron to remove wrinkles before waxing. If desired, you can finish the edges with a zigzag stitch, a serged edge, or simply by cutting the edges with pinking shears.

3. Place a piece of parchment paper on a baking sheet. Preheat the oven to 225°F.

4. Working with one piece of fabric at a time, place the fabric in a single layer on the baking sheet, on top of the parchment paper. Using the paintbrush, wipe the beeswax mixture onto the surface of the fabric. Place the baking sheet in the oven. Leave it only long enough to melt the beeswax. The beeswax mixture will melt into the fabric and spread. Once the fabric darkens and glistens, showing that the beeswax is fully melted, remove the baking sheet from the oven.

5. Use the paintbrush to make sure the beeswax mixture fully saturates the cloth. It may pool in some areas and leave other areas drier. Move the wax around the fabric, using the paintbrush as necessary. Blot excess wax using another piece of fabric, laid out over the first piece.

6. When the fabric is saturated with the wax mixture, flip the fabric over on the baking sheet, so that the blotting fabric is on

the bottom and takes the excess wax. Using your hands on the warmed fabric, work the excess wax into the less saturated areas of the fabric. Return the baking sheet to the oven, briefly, just long enough to liquefy the wax. Remove the first fabric from the baking sheet and drape over a clothes rack to dry.

7. The blotting fabric is now your working fabric. Use a brush to spread more of the beeswax mixture around on the fabric. Try to cover the fabric evenly with a thin layer of the wax mixture. Place the baking sheet in the oven to melt the wax. As soon as the wax is liquefied, remove the baking sheet from the oven. Spread the melted wax around with the paintbrush. Blot the excess wax from the working fabric using a new piece of fabric. Flip the fabric over so that the blotting fabric is now on the bottom. Return this briefly to the oven to re-liquefy. Remove the working fabric to a rack to dry.

8. Repeat with more squares of fabric, going through the process one at a time, and blotting the excess wax onto the next piece of fabric. Allow the beeswax-impregnated fabric squares to dry fully. Once dry, wipe both sides of each piece of fabric with a damp cloth to remove any residual wax or resin before using.

TO USE

The beeswax can be warmed in the hands and will conform to the shape of a bowl it is covering. Use it to wrap sandwiches. You can wrap snacks, vegetables, cheese, or even loaves of bread, provided that the pieces of fabric are large enough. The pine resin is naturally antimicrobial and adds strength, cling, and malleability to the mixture.

TO CLEAN

Wash in cool to warm water, using mild dish detergent. Hang to dry. Fold and store.

Do not machine wash. Do not wash in hot water.

Sandwich Wraps

While you could use the larger food wrap for wrapping lunch sandwiches, sometimes you want a smaller size for less bulk. These 10 x 10 beeswax wraps are the perfect size for sandwiches. This recipe omits the pine resin, since when you are wrapping sandwiches you don't need the wrap to cling. The formula is a little different but it still makes a flexible wrap. These wraps close with a button tie so that your sandwich won't escape on the bus.

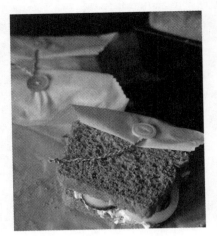

YIELD: 4 sandwich wraps

INGREDIENTS

3 tablespoons beeswax

1 tablespoon jojoba oil

4 10 x 10-inch squares quilting fabric

8 wooden buttons

4 10-inch pieces twine

DIRECTIONS

1. Melt the beeswax and jojoba oil together in a glass jar using a double boiler. Stir to make a smooth mixture.

2. Take a piece of fabric and follow steps 2 to 8 of Beeswax Food Wrap (page 167). Repeat these steps with each of the fabric squares.

3. When your wraps are fully dry, sew two wooden buttons onto two diagonal corners of each fabric. Tie a piece of twine around one of the buttons on each piece of fabric and secure the twine on the button with a wreath knot.

TO USE

Place your sandwich in the center of your wrap. Take one of the corners that doesn't have a button and cross it over the sandwich. Tuck the corner in under the bread. Take the opposite, button-less corner and wrap it over the sandwich from the other side. Tuck it under. Now take the two opposing corners that are left. Fold these to the center of your sandwich. Use the piece of twine to wrap around the two buttons, in a figure eight, to keep the sandwich wrap closed.

TO CLEAN

Wash in cool to warm water using mild dish detergent. Hang to dry. Fold and store.

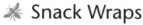 Snack Wraps

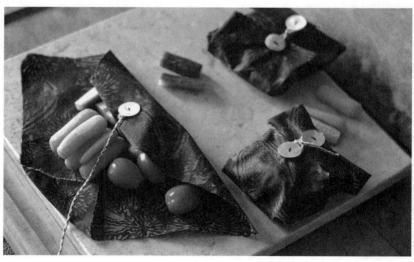

These are great little packets for cookies, veggie sticks, or cheese. They wrap using the same closure as the sandwich wraps, but in a smaller package for less bulk. When you open the snack wrap, you have a flat serving napkin to keep the food clean while you eat.

YIELD: 4 wraps

INGREDIENTS

2 tablespoons beeswax

2 teaspoons jojoba

2 tablespoons pine resin

4 8 x 8-inch 100% cotton quilting fabric pieces

Thread

8 half-inch buttons

4 yards butcher twine

DIRECTIONS

1. Follow the directions for the Beeswax Food Wraps (page 167).

2. When your wraps are fully dry, fold down two corners, diagonal from each other. Sew two half-inch buttons onto these corners for each wrap.

3. Take a 36-inch piece of twine and twist it clockwise between your thumb and forefinger, to increase the twist. Hold the end you are not twisting in your non-dominant hand. Keep twisting until the twine begins to double back on itself. Fold the twine in half to make a shorter piece of four-ply twine. The twine will spontaneously twist together. Tie a piece of 4-ply twine around one of the buttons on each piece of fabric, and secure the twine on the button with a wreath knot.

TO USE

Place your snack in the center of your wrap. Take one of the corners that doesn't have a button and cross it over the snack. Tuck the corner in under the snack. Take the opposite, button-less corner and wrap it over the snack from the other side. Tuck it under. Now take the two opposing corners that are left. Wrap the twine in a figure eight around both buttons to secure the snack inside the wrap.

✳ Cheese Wax

Waxing is used to preserve Gouda and other hard cheeses as they age. Cheese that is waxed does not need a humidity-controlled environment in order to age well. The wax prevents moisture loss.

Cheese waxes are available from dairy suppliers. These waxes are made of petroleum-based paraffin, microcrystalline wax, and chemical dyes. Beeswax is a natural alternative to petroleum-based waxes in cheesemaking. Its use contributes to the flavor of the aging cheese. Beeswax can be washed and reused, unlike petroleum-based cheese waxes that degrade over time, making beeswax an economical choice for home cheesemaking.

This recipe uses tallow because it has no scent and will not impart additional flavors to the cheese as it ages. This cheese wax is pliable and will conform to the shape of the cheese without cracking. The pine resin is antimicrobial.

Cheese that will be waxed before aging should be pressed in a cheese press. Only hard cheese should be waxed. Soft cheese contains too much moisture to age well when waxed, and may mold. Cheese rounds must be dry before waxing.

YIELD: Enough wax to dip 4 (2-pound) rounds of cheese

INGREDIENTS

1½ cups beeswax

½ cup tallow

1 teaspoon pine resin

DIRECTIONS

1. In a shallow pan at least 3 inches deep and large enough to dip the cheese rounds into, melt together the beeswax, tallow, and pine resin. Stir to integrate the pine resin with the melted beeswax. Allow to cool just enough that the wax remains melted.

2. The wax should be melted in a dedicated wax pot. The pot must be big enough and with sufficient wax in the pot to submerge the cheese a little more than halfway. Watch the wax to ensure that it doesn't overheat.

3. Dry the cheese rounds completely. Hold the cheese in two hands. Submerge it in the wax quickly and remove it. Hold it over the pan to allow the excess wax to drip back in. Place the cheese round to cool on a board until the wax is firm.

4. Flip the cheese round over and hold it by the waxed side with both hands. Quickly submerge the second side in the wax. Cool it again on the board. Repeat this waxing and cooling until both sides of the cheese have been dipped in the wax three times.

5. The cheese can be slippery during the dipping process. Take care that it doesn't slip out of your hands and cause the wax to splash. Should you inadvertently splash wax on your counter, allow the wax to cool. It should peel off without any problem.

Waxed cheese retains the moisture that cheese needs to thrive during the aging process. Keep it in a cool environment and flip it once a week as it ages. I store my waxed cheese in a sanitized plastic box with a tight-fitting lid in a cool pantry.

⚜ Beeswax Cast-Iron Seasoning

Use a bar of beeswax to season cast-iron cookware and preserve the finish.

YIELD: Seasoning for one frying pan

INGREDIENTS

1 2-ounce bar beeswax

DIRECTIONS

1. Heat your cleaned cast-iron pan in a 475°F oven for ten minutes. Remove the pan from the oven. Immediately slide a bar of beeswax over the surface of the frying pan, being sure to also

coat the sides of the pan. The pan is very hot. Wear a heatproof oven mitt to do this. Remove the excess wax with a paper towel.

2. Return the pan to the oven. Bake for one hour at 475°F. Turn off the oven and allow the pan to cool there until it is warm to the touch, but you can safely handle it.

3. Remove the pan from the oven and reapply the beeswax. Remove excess wax with a paper towel. Bake the pan for one hour at 475°F. Turn off the oven and allow the pan to cool.

4. Repeat this for each layer of beeswax until you have obtained the finish you desire on your cast iron. At 475°F, the beeswax forms a polymer film on the surface of the cast iron.

🐝 Air Freshener Wax Tarts

These wax tarts replace chemical room fresheners, promoting healthier indoor air. These are useful in the kitchen to remove dank odors without toxic chemicals. Each wax tart is about 1½ ounces. This project includes three homey scents: citrus, calm, and alert.

YIELD: 5 wax tarts

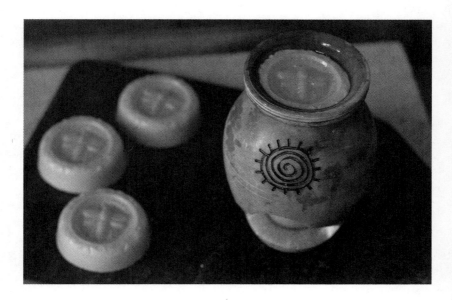

INGREDIENTS

½ cup beeswax

½ cup cocoa butter

½ teaspoon sweet orange essential oil

1 teaspoon bergamot essential oil

1 teaspoon lemon verbena essential oil

DIRECTIONS

1. Make a double boiler with a glass measuring cup. Place beeswax and cocoa butter in the cup. Melt them together over medium heat. Once the wax has melted, stir and add the essential oils.

2. Prepare molds. If you are using silicone molds, the wax tarts will pop out. If you are using a plastic mold, apply silicone mold release spray to the mold before you fill it with the beeswax mixture. Pour the mixture into the mold and allow it to harden at room temperature.

3. Remove the wax tarts from the mold. Store in a jar with a tight-fitting lid to preserve the fragrance.

TO USE

Place the wax tart into the top of an essential oil candle diffuser. Light a tea light candle below the reservoir. As the wax in the reservoir melts, it will release its scent. You can refresh the scent of the wax tart by adding more essential oils to the reservoir when the fragrance dims. The wax tart can be reused over and over.

When you are ready to clean the reservoir, simply warm the dish and wipe out the used wax. The wax mixture can be reused in other applications, if desired. There is no waste.

VARIATIONS

Follow the instructions for the above recipe, but substitute with the following essential oils.

Calm

1 teaspoon lavender essential oil

½ teaspoon marjoram essential oil

½ teaspoon rosemary essential oil

Alert

1 teaspoon peppermint essential oil

1 teaspoon rosemary essential oil

½ teaspoon eucalyptus essential oil

Beeswax in the Workshop and Garage

Beeswax is an integral element in the workshop. You've already seen how helpful it can be as a polish and preservative in other areas of your home. In the workshop it can also be used as a lubricant, a sealant, and an ingredient in adhesives. For more ideas for utilizing beeswax in the workshop and garage, check out the Chapter 7, Beeswax in the Garden, and Chapter 8, Beeswax for Sport and Leisure.

🐝 Sealing Putty

Sealing putty is used to fill cracks and seal plumbing joints.

YIELD: 1 (6-ounce) container

INGREDIENTS

2 teaspoons beeswax

¼ cup raw flax-seed oil

2 tablespoons calcium carbonate

DIRECTIONS

1. Melt the beeswax in a glass jar in a double boiler. Stir in raw flaxseed oil and continue heating until the beeswax and flaxseed

oil can be stirred together into a smooth mixture. Remove from heat. Allow the mixture to cool to room temperature.

2. Gradually add calcium carbonate, 1 tablespoon at a time, creating a smooth, stiff paste that pulls away from the sides of the jar. Knead the paste, adding more calcium carbonate until a stiff putty texture is obtained.

3. Store this in an airtight container with a resealable lid.

Just a Bar of Wax

There are loads of things that can be done in the home and workshop with just a bar of wax:

* Dip wine bottle tops in melted beeswax to finish the seals and keep the corks from shrinking.

* Lubricate hinges to stop the squeak.

* Lubricate drawer edges or glides to make them glide smoothly.

* Lubricate screws before turning them into wood to prevent the wood from splitting.

* Coat metal tools in high humidity areas to prevent corrosion.

* Coat sewing thread to make it stronger and resist tangling and knotting.

* Use it as hot glue for temporary hold.

* Use it at the wood lathe to reduce sanding dust.

* Give a satin finish to hand-turned wood. Apply it directly at the lathe. The friction from the turning melts just enough wax to finish the piece.

* Dab some on the screw chuck when turning green wood to make it easier to remove the wood after turning.

* Use it on the bottom of woodworking planes to smooth the bottom, reduce friction, and protect from rust.

✳ Workshop Hot Glue

This glue is an age-old recipe that has been used by knife makers to fasten steel blades to wooden knife handles and by ancient civilizations to fasten arrowheads to shafts. It can be used in any application to bond metal to wood or wood to wood. Since it must be worked hot, it is not suitable for bonding to plastic. This recipe can be doubled or tripled, keeping the ratios the same.

YIELD: 1 (1½-ounce) tin

INGREDIENTS

1 tablespoon pine resin

1 teaspoon beeswax

½ teaspoon iron oxide powder

DIRECTIONS

1. Make a double boiler in a tin can. Melt the pine resin over medium heat. When the pine resin is liquid, stir in the beeswax. Continue stirring until the beeswax is melted and mixed with the pine resin.

2. Add the iron oxide powder and stir to mix. If the iron oxide is not available to you, ocher, brick dust, clay, or finely powdered charcoal can be used in place of iron oxide.

3. Use the glue while it is hot. Store in a tin with a tight-fitting lid. Remove the lid to reheat.

TO USE

Using a stick or dauber brush, coat the metal or wood that you wish to glue. Apply to one piece only. Immediately press the second piece onto the glued piece and wipe off excess glue. Clamp together until firm.

This glue can be reheated to use again; however, do not overheat. Overheating breaks the adhesive bonds and reduces the strength of the bond. Avoid getting steam in the tin.

For an adhesive with half the holding power, omit the iron oxide and increase the beeswax to 1 tablespoon. Apply the glue hot. Clamp together until firm.

🐝 Car Wax

You don't need to buy commercial car wax and polish to protect your car's shine and finish. This polish lasts longer than commercial products and is more eco-friendly, too. When applied correctly and allowed to cure before buffing, this has water-repelling properties similar to commercial waxes that contain toxic solvents and dryers.

The addition of carnauba wax gives this car wax a very tough shine, filling in scratches. Buff until the surface gleams and there are no streaks. Wax may be reapplied to build up several layers of shine and protection.

YIELD: 3 (2-ounce) tins

INGREDIENTS

1 tablespoon beeswax granules

2 tablespoons carnauba wax granules

2 tablespoons raw flax oil

1 tablespoon orange wax

4 tablespoons d-limonene

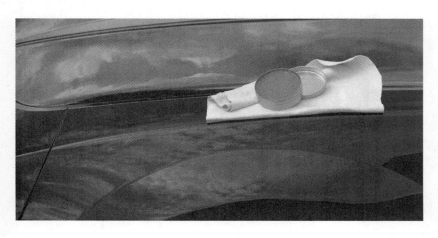

DIRECTIONS

1. Make a double boiler using a glass measuring cup. Melt together the beeswax, carnauba wax, flax oil, and orange wax over medium heat.

2. When the mixture is fully melted, stir in the d-limonene. Continue stirring until the mixture is completely liquid. Remove from the heat.

3. Pour into tins. Cool completely before using. Label.

TO USE

Wash your car and let it dry naturally. Using a soft, lint-free cloth, dip into the wax in the jar. Brush onto the car in a circular motion. Allow the wax to dry for about 10 or 15 minutes, or until the wax cures. Using a second dry cloth, buff the excess wax off the car.

Wax coating may be repeated to enhance its water-repelling qualities and shine.

Chapter 7

BEESWAX IN THE GARDEN

*To forget how to dig the earth and to
tend the soil is to forget ourselves.*

—Mahatma Gandhi

Beeswax is a natural adjunct to organic gardening. While water helps the garden to grow, moisture and mildew harm garden tools, equipment, and structures. Beeswax, with its water-repelling and sealing properties, can perform many tasks in the garden.

While many garden finishing and protective products contain petrochemicals and plastics, beeswax is a natural alternative that won't leave behind toxic residues in your soil. Impervious to water, beeswax protects against water damage and rot longer than many commercial products because it doesn't break down over time. It isn't damaged by sunlight. However, in applications that will be exposed to heat over 100°F, beeswax may become sticky and more malleable. This quality can be modified by reducing the percentage of beeswax in the formula.

Beeswax Protection for Garden Tools

Garden tools don't always make it back to the shed before the rain comes. Even worse is when you find the pruning shears on the ground after the snow melts in spring. No one plans to leave their tools out to get damaged by moisture, but when it happens, beeswax can help protect those expensive tools from rust.

The first step is to clean up any rust deposits on the tool blade. The easiest way to remove rust is to apply a paste of salt and vinegar. Apply it over the metal area of the tool and let it sit for 15 minutes. If the tool is heavily corroded, you can leave this salt and vinegar paste on the tool overnight. Using steel wool, rub the tool in a circular motion to remove corrosion. On heavily corroded tools, you may need to repeat the vinegar–salt paste application to remove all the rust.

Rinse and dry the tool fully before applying this beeswax preservative.

🐝 Metal Preservative

Beeswax provides a moisture barrier, preventing rust and corrosion when used regularly on garden tools.

YIELD: 1 (10-ounce) jar

INGREDIENTS

¼ cup beeswax

1 cup hemp seed oil

DIRECTIONS

1. Make a double boiler with a glass measuring cup. Melt the beeswax. Add the hemp seed oil and stir until the beeswax and oil are fully blended.

2. Store in a pint jar with a tight–fitting lid.

3. Apply this mixture to dry tool heads with a soft cloth. Allow this to dry on the tools overnight. Buff the tool lightly to remove the tackiness of the wax.

🐝 Tool Handle Preservative

Once the tool heads are free of rust and preserved, you don't want to let their wooden handles lose their strength. Tool handles left out in the elements dry out and the wood can split. Prevent this by applying a penetrating wax finish to the handles at the beginning and end of the growing season.

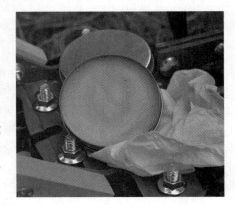

YIELD: 2 (3-ounce) tins

INGREDIENTS

¼ cup beeswax

¼ cup raw flax oil

¼ cup d–limonene

DIRECTIONS

1. Make a double boiler with a glass measuring cup. Melt the beeswax. Stir in raw the flax oil and continue stirring until the mixture is fully liquid. Remove the pan from the heat.

2. Stir in the d–limonene.

3. Store this preservative in two 3-ounce tins with tight-fitting lids.

TO USE

Lightly sand the tool handles if necessary to remove any splinters. Apply a light, even coating of the tool handle preservative with a paper towel. Wipe off any excess. Allow it to cure for 24 hours. Reapply a second coating of the preservative. Wipe off any excess. Wait an additional 24 hours before using the tool. Reapply a single coat of the preservative twice a year, in the spring and fall, in order to protect your tool handles from moisture. Allow this to dry for 24 hours before using the tool.

Protection for Your Outdoor Wooden Structures

The hardscape areas of your garden are subject to the weather all year round. They don't get put away at the end of the season. Wood exposed to the elements with no protection breaks down with exposure to ultraviolet light, fungi, and moisture.

Building the hardscape elements of your landscape with wood that is resistant to fungi and termites can prolong the life of your structures. Sealing wood with beeswax can further extend the life expectancy of wooden structures. The best woods for outdoor structures are wood types that are naturally resistant to fungi and termites.

Exceptionally resistant

* Black locust
* Red mulberry
* Osage orange
* Pacific yew

Very resistant

* Old-growth cypress
* Old-growth redwood
* White oak
* Cedar
* Mahogany
* Teak
* Black cherry
* Chestnut
* Juniper
* Honey locust
* Sassafras
* Black walnut

Moderately resistant

* Second growth cypress
* Douglas fir
* Larch

Use Beeswax Instead of WD-40

Beeswax acts as a penetrant, like WD-40. Sometimes two parts of a tool will rust together and you won't be able to separate them. To separate them, heat the metal parts of the tool. Apply beeswax to the heated tool so that it drips into the gap between the two parts. This will allow the pieces to slide apart.

🐝 Nontoxic Wood Sealant for Raised Garden Beds

Preserving the wood used to enclose raised garden beds is a conundrum. Popular wood preservatives contain toxic heavy metals that leach into the soil of a vegetable garden, potentially contaminating the soil and any food growing there. But because garden boxes are exposed to the weather and remain perpetually damp, some kind of preservative is necessary. Without a wood preservative, these garden beds need to be rebuilt with new wood every three or four years.

This nontoxic, beeswax–based wood preservative will extend the life of wooden garden beds without contaminating your soil. It forms a barrier that prevents rot–causing moisture from seeping into the wood. While it won't make your garden beds last forever, it will certainly extend their lifespan. This recipe can be doubled to cover larger garden projects.

This recipe is a messy one. Spread newspaper over your work area before you begin. You can use activated charcoal, but you can also use charcoal you saved from the campfire or woodstove. It can be messy pulverizing charcoal, though, so plan to do this part outdoors. To pulverize the charcoal, put it in a bag to contain it and then pound it to a powder with a mallet or vegetable pounder. Sift the charcoal and use the fine powder in this recipe. Conserve the large pieces for another purpose.

YIELD: 1 (10-ounce) jar

INGREDIENTS

¼ cup beeswax

1 cup walnut oil

2 tablespoons finely ground wood charcoal

DIRECTIONS

1. Create a double boiler using a glass measuring cup. Place the beeswax and walnut oil in the cup. Melt them together over medium heat.

2. Once the beeswax is fully melted, carefully stir in the charcoal. Continue stirring until the mixture is of a smooth consistency and there are no large globs of charcoal.

3. Store in a wide-mouth pint jar with a tight-fitting lid.

TO USE

Apply the paste mixture with a cloth or steel wool to all sides of new boards before you build your raised beds. Allow this to dry fully. Reapply in 24 hours.

Preservative and Sealant for Wicker Garden Furniture

Much of the garden furniture today is made of plastic rather than wood. If you are lucky enough to have a set of old-fashioned wicker or bent willow garden furniture, you can use this recipe to keep it in top shape.

YIELD: 1 (12-ounce) jar

INGREDIENTS

½ cup beeswax

½ cup grape seed oil

½ cup gum turpentine

1. Make a double boiler using a tin can. Add the beeswax and grape seed oil to the can. Melt over medium heat. Remove the pan from the heat.

2. Stir in the gum turpentine and continue stirring until a smooth paste forms.

3. Pour into a wide mouth pint jar with a tight-fitting lid.

TO USE

Apply this mixture with a soft cloth to the clean, dry surface of your wicker garden furniture. Be sure to get into the crevices between the wicker-work to form a protective seal. Allow the mixture to dry overnight. Reapply in 24 hours. Buff with a dry, lint-free cloth to remove any excess wax mixture.

🦟 Wood Preservative and Sealant for Fence Posts

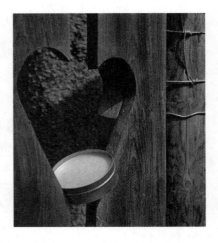

Fence posts are one of the more frustrating parts of the garden. Most pressure-treated fence posts leach heavy metal salts like arsenic and lead into the garden, potentially contaminating the soil. Untreated fence posts only last two or three years before they rot out at ground level. But finding a nontoxic wood preservative that is safe below the ground is a challenge.

The ideal wood preservative would provide a vapor barrier to keep moisture from entering the wood during high humidity. It would also condition the wood and prevent it from drying out and cracking. Ideally, it would provide a flexible finish that wouldn't flake off as the wood cells move and breathe.

YIELD: 1 (5–ounce) jar

INGREDIENTS

2 cups beeswax

2 cups raw flaxseed oil

½ cup pine rosin

2 cups d-limonene

¼ cup boric acid powder

DIRECTIONS

1. Melt the beeswax and flaxseed oil in a tin can in a water bath. In a separate tin can, warm up the pine rosin to liquefy it. Pour the pine rosin into the beeswax, stirring while you add it. Remove the pan from the heat source.

2. Add the d-limonene to the beeswax mixture while stirring constantly.

3. Stir in the boric acid powder, removing any clumps.

4. Pour into a wide-mouth glass jar with a tight-fitting lid.

TO USE

Paint the portion of the fence post that will be underground with the beeswax preservative. Allow the mixture to dry on the fence post overnight. Wipe off the excess. Reapply in 24 hours, when the treated wood is dry to the touch.

Beeswax for Propagation

Beeswax is naturally antimicrobial due to the minute amounts of residual propolis that remain in the wax. This, plus the malleability of beeswax, make it an ideal wax for grafting and sealing wounds in trees. Both orchardists and mushroom growers rely on beeswax for the success of their propagation.

✳ Grafting Wax

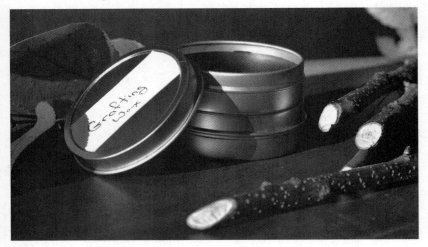

Grafting wax is used in the orchard to seal new grafts on fruit trees. It prevents moisture loss and bacterial contamination while the new fruit wood bonds with the rooting stalk, forming a single tree. The addition of charcoal protects the new graft from sunlight while the graft is taking.

YIELD: 1 (16-ounce) tin

INGREDIENTS

½ cup beeswax

½ cup tallow

1 cup of pine resin

2 tablespoons powdered charcoal

¼ cup gum turpentine

DIRECTIONS

1. Make a double boiler using a tin can. Place the beeswax and tallow in the can. Melt them together over medium heat. In a separate can, heat the pine resin until it is liquid. Thoroughly stir the warmed, liquid pine resin into the beeswax mixture to make a smooth mixture.

2. Remove from the heat and stir in powdered charcoal. Continue stirring until the mixture is of a smooth consistency.

3. Allow this to cool to about 100°F. Stir in the gum turpentine. Continue stirring the mixture until it is smooth.

4. Pour into tin. Cap tightly.

TO USE

Use your fingers to mold the grafting wax on grafts. The grafting wax will harden as it dries, forming a protective barrier for the tree.

🐝 Beeswax Seal for Mushroom Logs

When inoculating freshly sawn logs with mushroom mycelium for growing shiitake or oyster mushrooms, the holes in the logs must be sealed to allow the mycelium to run without competition from microbes or other fungi. Waxing also seals in moisture while sealing out parasites. Because beeswax has a low melting temperature, it is often used for mushroom culture. This requires a camp stove set up outside to keep the wax liquid while the logs are being plugged with mushroom spawn.

One drawback to simply dripping 100 percent beeswax over the spawn plug is that the wax shrinks as it cools, leaving a brittle button of wax on the bark of the tree that may not fully cover the plug. It's quite common for wax seals to fall off in the year it takes the mycelium to run throughout the wood.

This recipe is less brittle than pure beeswax, and more durable. You'll still need to warm the mixture in order to apply it.

YIELD: Enough wax for 50 to 60 mushroom plugs

INGREDIENTS

1 cup beeswax

¼ cup tallow

1 tablespoon pine pitch

DIRECTIONS

1. Create a double boiler using a tin can. Place the beeswax and tallow in the can and melt them together over medium heat.

2. Stir in the pine pitch and continue heating until the pine pitch is blended into the wax mixture. Stir to mix in the pine pitch with the wax mixture. Remove from the heat.

3. This can be stored in the can until you are ready to use it.

TO USE

Melt the beeswax seal over medium heat in a water bath. Brush over the mushroom plugs during mushroom log cultivation to seal the plug holes.

Beeswax Waterproofing in the Garden

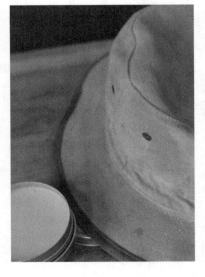

While traditional recipes for oil cloth include toxic chemicals, gardening requires gentler scented waterproofing. When wearing waterproof hats and shoes, you don't want to absorb the heavy metals used in petroleum distillates through your skin. Furthermore, when the waterproofing comes in contact with your garden produce, you need to be a little more discriminating. No one wants to lay their fresh, organic lettuce in a gathering basket reeking of boiled linseed oil and turpentine distillates. Thankfully, with the following beeswax recipes, you can choose organic waterproofing products for these sensitive applications.

Waterproof Shade Hat

How many times has it started to rain right when you needed to run out to the garden to grab some herbs? When your wide-brimmed hat is an oilskin hat, the rain won't faze you. This waterproofing formula is a variation on the traditional, without the cadmium, lead, and petroleum. As an added bonus, the lingering citrus scent will repel blood-sucking insects.

YIELD: 1 (4-ounce) tin

INGREDIENTS

2 tablespoons hemp seed oil

¼ cup beeswax

2 tablespoons d-limonene

DIRECTIONS

1. Create a double boiler with a glass measuring cup. Simmer the hemp seed oil until a skin begins to form on the surface of the oil.

2. Stir in the beeswax. Continue simmering until the beeswax is fully melted. Stir to incorporate the hemp seed oil and the beeswax. Remove from the heat.

3. Stir in the d-limonene and continue stirring until the mixture is smooth.

4. Pour into a 4-ounce tin. You can use this mixture interchangeably with any other waterproofing recipe in this chapter.

TO USE

Wash and dry the hat to remove any dirt or sizing. Apply the paste using a stiff brush or cloth, working the wax deeply into the surface of the fabric. Apply a thin, even layer of wax. If you get too much wax in one area, use your brush to move it around.

You only want to coat the outside of the fabric, leaving the surface next to your skin free of the waterproofing.

Now, use a hair dryer to gently warm the wax and allow it to penetrate and bond with the fabric.

To clean the waterproof fabric, wipe with a damp cloth. Do not wash the fabric in the washing machine after it is waxed.

🐝 Waterproof Canvas Hammock, Awning, or Chair Fabric

Canvas garden furniture can be weatherproofed with this beeswax application. By waterproofing the surface of canvas that is exposed to the elements, you will extend its life. Once the fabric is waterproofed and cured, water will bead off the surface rather than being absorbed. The waterproofing can be reapplied as needed without harming the integrity of the canvas fabric.

YIELD: 1 (5 ounce) bar

INGREDIENTS

¼ cup of beeswax

1 tablespoon pine resin

2 tablespoons lanolin

¼ cup jojoba oil

DIRECTIONS

1. Make a double boiler using a tin can. Place the beeswax in the can and melt over medium heat. In a separate can, heat the pine resin in the same water bath.

2. Stir the lanolin into the beeswax until the mixture is smooth. Stir the jojoba oil into the beeswax mixture and continue stirring until it is thoroughly blended.

3. Add the melted pine resin to the beeswax mixture and continue stirring to completely mix it. The pine resin has a tendency to sink to the bottom, so you'll want to scrape the bottom of the tin as you stir.

4. Remove from the heat and allow it to cool slightly, stirring as it cools. While it is still liquid, pour the mixture into a 5-ounce silicone bar mold. Allow the bar to cool completely. Wrap in brown paper to keep your hands clean while using it.

TO USE

Wash and dry 100 percent cotton, linen, or hemp fabric. Iron to remove wrinkles. Apply in an inconspicuous area of the fabric to ensure that you like the effect of the waterproofing.

Wax the outside of the garment as desired.

Apply the waterproofing bar by rubbing the bar into the surface of the fabric in long, even strokes. Overlap each stroke so that there are no empty spots on the surface of the fabric. Use your hands to move the wax coating around the surface of the fabric to ensure an even coat.

Once you are satisfied with the way your canvas fabric looks, you can hang it up to cure. After 24 to 48 hours it will lose its tackiness and be ready to use.

TO CLEAN

Wipe with a damp cloth on the surface of the canvas. Do not put the fabric in your washing machine. The wax coating will ruin your washing machine and could clog your drains.

The wax coating will repel dirt and stains and can be renewed as often as necessary to maintain the oilskin finish.

🐝 Waterproof Shoes

Waterproof your shoes with this blend and keep your feet dry when you slip your canvas shoes on to run out to the garden.

YIELD: 3 (2-ounce) tins

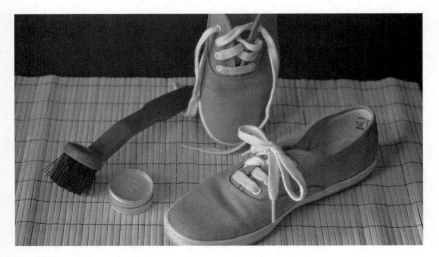

INGREDIENTS

2 tablespoons beeswax

1 teaspoon carnauba wax

2 tablespoons grape seed oil

1 teaspoon pine resin

1 tablespoon d–limonene

DIRECTIONS

1. Create a double boiler using a tin can. Warm the beeswax, carnauba wax, and grape seed oil together in the tin can until the beeswax is melted.

2. In a separate tin, warm the pine resin until it is liquid. Pour the warmed pine resin into the beeswax mixture. Stir until the mixture is uniform.

3. Stir in the d–limonene and remove from the heat. Stir the mixture while it cools so that the beeswax doesn't clump. When it gets thick, pour into tins.

TO USE

Wash and thoroughly dry a pair of canvas shoes. Stuff the shoes with newspaper to help them hold their shape during the waxing process and to absorb any excess wax. Using a brush or dauber, brush the beeswax mixture onto the surface of the shoes. Apply a thin, even coating. Using a hair dryer, warm the beeswax coating until it glistens. This will drive the waterproof coating deeper into the fibers of the shoe, filling in any gaps within the canvas weave. Allow to cool and set overnight before wearing.

TO CLEAN

Wipe with a damp cloth. Shoes may be washed by hand in cool water and allowed to dry away from a heat source. Do not put in the washing machine.

Repeat the waterproofing treatment as the shoes lose their water resistance.

Sealant and Waterproofing for Baskets

Most purchased wicker baskets have a shellac finish. The finish protects the structure of the basket and improves its durability. Over time this shellac finish can wear off, leaving your favorite gathering basket susceptible to the elements. Sealing the basket with beeswax can increase its effective lifespan.

YIELD: 3 (2-ounce) tins

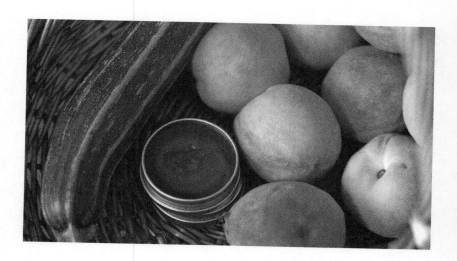

INGREDIENTS

3 tablespoons walnut oil

¼ cup beeswax

2 tablespoons orange wax

2 tablespoons d–limonene

DIRECTIONS

1. Create a double boiler using a tin can in a pot of water. In the tin can, heat walnut oil until a skin begins to form on the surface.

2. Stir in the beeswax and simmer until it melts.

3. Add the orange wax. Stir while adding the d–limonene, until the mixture is smooth. Remove from the heat.

4. Pour into tins.

TO USE

Apply the mixture with a soft cloth, being sure to get it into the crevices of the basket. Allow the mixture to sit on the basket for one hour. Wipe excess off with a dry, lint-free cloth. Apply as many coats as you like, wiping off any excess sealant between coats.

Allow at least 24 hours for the sealant to cure before using the basket.

Bees in the Garden

A chapter on using beeswax in the garden wouldn't be complete without talking about bees in the garden. Bees are an important part of your gardening success. Without pollinators, your fruit trees and many of your vegetable plants wouldn't produce any fruit at all. There are many native bees that pollinate more efficiently than honey bees, but *Apis mellifera,* the western honeybee, is the most common bee that produces honey and wax, as well as pollination.

My beekeeper friends tell me that they get around 60 to 80 pounds of honey per beehive, while still leaving the bees ample honey to get through the winter. The estimated wax yield is 1 to 2 pounds of beeswax per hive. While it doesn't sound like a lot of beeswax, there are 3.3 million beehives in the US and Canada, at this writing. Most backyard beekeepers have two or three colonies by the end of summer. Watching the bees is fascinating.

Raising Honey Bees in Your Garden

Putting up a beehive is just like putting up a birdhouse or a bat house. You'll just need some lumber and a few carpentry skills to make a hive that is fit for a queen bee.

During the spring and summer, when bees are actively collecting nectar and making honey, hives can get too crowded. When this happens, a maiden queen will often fly off with a portion of the hive looking for a new home. When bees swarm, they are looking for a new hive. If you have a hive waiting for them, they might just pick your hive to live in. When you catch a swarm, you catch a strong hive, because only strong hives swarm.

The presence and aroma of beeswax is a natural attractant to honeybees. If you are hoping to catch a hive of bees for your garden, building a hive box and sealing it with a natural beeswax-based sealant is a very good way to attract a swarm. Use any of the wood sealants in this chapter to make your hive box weatherproof while still allowing it to breathe.

A Warré hive is easy to build from materials you have on hand. You can build one for under $30. For more information on attracting honeybees, including woodworking plans for a Warré hive, see the Resources on page 278.

🐝 Bee Swarm Lure

If you want to increase your chance of successfully attracting a swarm, you can add an attractant to your bait hive. Lemongrass is very similar to the queen bee's scent. Honeybees find the mixture of lemongrass and beeswax irresistible.

YIELD: 3 ounces

INGREDIENTS

2 tablespoons beeswax

¼ cup olive oil

40 drops (2 milliliters) lemongrass essential oil

DIRECTIONS

1. Make a double boiler using a tin can. Melt the beeswax and olive oil together in the can, over medium heat. Remove from the heat.

2. Add the lemongrass essential oil. Stir the mixture while it cools, just until it begins to thicken. Pour into a 4-ounce tin. Allow the lure to cool.

TO USE

Smear 1 tablespoon of the swarm lure at the back of the hive box. Set the hive box in the shade, raised above the ground where it is dry. Wait for the bees to swarm. You just might get lucky and catch your own perpetual source of beeswax and honey while you help the bees survive.

Chapter 8

BEESWAX FOR SPORT AND LEISURE

He is not worthy of the honey-comb that shuns
the hives because the bees have stings.

—William Shakespeare

The protective and conditioning qualities of beeswax make it a natural help for sports and leisure equipment and supplies. Whether you find your fun beside a campfire, in reenactment events, at the rodeo, at the range, or out on the slopes, beeswax provides protection, waterproofing, lubricity, and even fuel to keep you dry, comfortable, and enjoying your sport.

No one plans to cause a negative environmental impact when they are having fun, but many common sports products do exactly that. Petrochemicals left by hikers and campers leave their carbon footprint in the back country. Chemical sunscreen is implicated in the rapid destruction of the coral reef. The chemicals in commonly used ski waxes are causing permanent damage to the watersheds around ski country. With these beeswax alternatives to common products, you won't be "that guy."

Camping

I have the worst of luck camping. As a homeschool family, we always thought we'd beat the rush and get our summer camping trip in before July. On our worst camping year ever, we camped in Kootenay National Park in the Rocky Mountains. We drove all night with three sleeping children and waited at the park kiosk till they opened at 7:30 a.m. We set up the two-room tent and took turns sleeping and watching the kids. We'd planned to stay five nights. Then the rain started. It poured. It thundered. At 3 a.m., lightning hit the park's transformer and the power went out. The campground was evacuated. We drove on to Edmonton the next day and camped at a private campground. We stayed one night, but the rain followed us.

"We'll go to Drumheller in the desert," we thought. "It won't rain in the desert." We drove for hours, getting to Drumheller as the sun set. We put the tent up by camp lantern. We struggled to get a fire going so we could dry out our wet clothes. Before we even crawled into our sleeping bags, the rain started. The next day, we packed up our soaked tent, sleeping bags, and gear and drove for 12 hours home to Vancouver. Our two-week vacation was shortened to three nights.

I needed beeswax in those days. Camping trips would have been happier if we'd only known then what we know now.

❋ Waterproof Tents and Tarps

Do you remember the old canvas army tents? Remember that distinctive acrid smell? That was the perfume of boiled linseed oil and petroleum distillates. You don't need to create that pungent scent when you make your own canvas waterproofing.

This recipe will work on heavy tent canvas and tarps. You can double or triple the recipe so you don't run out on active jobs. The d-limonene will repel mosquitoes and biting insects, keeping them away from your gear, too.

This can be reapplied on an annual basis to keep your gear water-proof. Allow your tents and tarps to dry thoroughly in the sunlight before putting them away for the season.

YIELD: 3 cups

INGREDIENTS

1⅓ cups beeswax

1⅓ cups raw flaxseed oil

½ cup d-limonene

DIRECTIONS

1. Make a double boiler using a tin can. Simmer the beeswax and raw flaxseed oil in the can on medium heat until the beeswax melts. Stir to blend well.

2. Pour in the d-limonene while stirring. Mix until well blended. Remove from the heat. Continue stirring while the mixture cools. It will thicken slightly but remain pourable.

3. When it is cool enough to handle, spoon into a 1-quart glass jar. A peanut butter jar or similar container will let you get a paintbrush into the container without a mess.

TO USE

Wash canvas with soap and water. Dry completely. Spread the tent or tarp so that it is upright and stretched and there are no folds that could result in an uneven application. Paint the waterproofing on the canvas fabric evenly. Using a hair dryer or heat gun, heat the fabric to allow the beeswax to permeate deeply into the threads, forming a strong bond. Apply a second coat after the first coat has dried. When the cloth has enough coats, water will bead off it without being absorbed. Allow this to cure for 48 hours before using the tent in the rain.

✳ Solid Waterproofing Bar

Before there were Teflon boots and Gore-Tex® jackets, there was oil cloth. Oilcloth was the waterproof fabric used by fishermen, sailors, woodsmen, and cowboys to keep the weather out. Yellow and smelling strongly of turpentine, oil cloth was hard wearing and dependable in wet, windy conditions. Today, waxed outdoor clothing is making a resurgence.

This waxing bar is used as a waterproofing treatment for both leather and cloth. It is applied as a solid wax, making it very convenient for trekking or traveling. There are several commercial products that use paraffin wax or combinations of paraffin and beeswax in their "secret" waterproofing formulas. Some are sold as creams that can be applied by rubbing into the fabric, like a shoe polish. Others come in a solid bar that is applied by rubbing the bar directly onto the fabric and curing with the heat from an iron or heat gun.

You can manipulate the stiffness, breathability, flexibility, and durability of the fabric with the number of layers of wax you apply to the cloth. A more flexible, more breathable, but less durable and not-quite-so-waterproof cloth results with only one or two applications. Get a more complete waterproofing, with a stiffer, less breathable, but more durable fabric by adding more layers of the waxing compound.

Expect to reapply the wax after three or four washings. Garments and cloth treated with a solid waterproofing bar may be washed in cold water, by hand, and hung to dry.

Waxing will darken the color of the fabric and give it a light sheen. Test your garment in an inconspicuous spot before waxing the whole garment.

The best fabric candidates for waterproofing are tightly woven 100 percent cotton, hemp, or linen. Denim is a more loosely woven fabric and tends to feel heavy when waterproofed with wax.

Likely candidates for waxing include picnic table cloths, tents, tarps, aprons, painter's drop cloths, artist's smocks, baby bibs, canvas jackets, canvas hats, and canvas shoes.

YIELD: 1 (5-ounce) bar

INGREDIENTS

2 tablespoons carnauba wax

2 tablespoons raw flaxseed oil

4 tablespoons beeswax

2 teaspoons d-limonene

DIRECTIONS

1. Create a double boiler using a tin can. Simmer the carnauba wax and flaxseed oil in the can over medium heat until the wax melts.

2. Add the beeswax and continue simmering until it melts. Remove from the heat.

3. While stirring the mixture, add the d-limonene. Continue stirring to fully combine.

4. Pour into a 5-ounce silicone bar mold.

5. Cool the bar completely. Remove from the mold. Allow the bar to cure and the wax to recrystallize before using. Usually overnight is sufficient; 72 hours is best.

TO USE

Rub the bar of wax onto your garment using long strokes. Apply in a thin but even coat. Using a clothes iron set on polyester, iron the garment to cause the wax to penetrate into the fibers. Blot excess wax from the fabric with paper. Alternatively, set the wax into the fabric with a heat gun, being careful not to burn the fabric. For increased waterproofing, add a second or even a third coat. The fabric will be dry to the touch and slightly darker in color. It will be a little stiffer, too. Allow the fabric to dry fully before wearing.

Clothing treated with this solid wax bar will be waterproof and wind resistant.

✼ Waterproof Matches

I have had my share of trying to start a fire in a drizzle. It only takes a couple of minutes out in the rain to wreck a whole box of matches. In the wind, your lighter is useless, too. These waterproof matches can be kept in a tin along with a couple pieces of char cloth for those days when the kindling is wet and the fire just won't start.

You'll need wooden matchsticks. You can use strike-on-the-box matches or strike-anywhere matches. If you are using strike-on-the-box matches, you'll need the edge of the match box, so keep it dry as well.

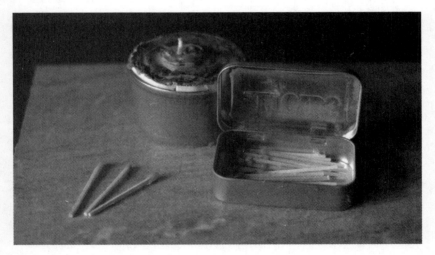

YIELD: 25 waterproof matches

MATERIALS

Small amount of beeswax

1 box of wooden matchsticks

DIRECTIONS

1. Create a double boiler using a small tin can. Add the beeswax to the can and melt over medium heat.

2. Dip the matches into the wax, just deep enough to cover the strike head.

3. Lay the matches on top of the match box, allowing the match heads to overhang the box.

4. Allow the match heads to dry. This only takes a minute or two.

5. Store the waterproof matches in a tin box. Add a couple pieces of char cloth and a strike card to your kit.

TO USE

Scrape the wax off the head of the match with your fingernail. Strike the match against the strike card from the box of matches. If you are using strike-anywhere matches, you'll need a strike surface to provide adequate friction.

Backpacker/Emergency Single-Use Stove

Living in the mountains, we are always prepared for winter driving conditions. I keep an emergency candle stove in the car, just in case. Beeswax is a better fuel for use in an enclosed space, as beeswax doesn't give off toxic fumes as it burns the way solid fuel stoves and paraffin candles do.

When in use, the can will get very hot, and you'll need a noncombustible surface to set it on.

You can use this stove with a 3-pound can to make a cooking surface. It will also provide quite a bit of heat in an enclosed space. Take the usual precautions around an open flame when using this stove in an enclosed space or around pets or children. Provide ventilation.

To make this, you'll need a small, flat can, like a 7-ounce salmon or tuna can. The quality of the beeswax isn't as important in this project.

Use the waste beeswax after filtering your wax for candlemaking or cosmetics.

YIELD: 1 solid fuel stove/burner

MATERIALS

Empty 7-ounce can

Several corrugated cardboard strips

3 prepared wicks and wick tabs

Bobby pins

1 cup beeswax

DIRECTIONS

1. Clean and remove the label from the can. Cut the corrugated cardboard into strips the same width as the can is high. You'll need enough strips to fill the can.

2. Roll the strips of corrugated cardboard in a tight roll and place them inside the can, long side down.

3. Insert wicks, with wick tabs equidistant around the inside of the can. Support the wicks upright using bobby pins.

4. Make a double boiler using a tin can. Add the beeswax to the can and melt over medium heat. Pour the melted wax over the cardboard in the prepared can. Allow the cardboard to absorb the beeswax. Add more beeswax to fill in any areas that got less beeswax in the first pour. Correct the wick position if necessary, while the wax is still soft.

5. Allow the single-use stove to cure for 48 hours before using.

TO USE

Place the stove on a noncombustible, stable surface. Light the wicks on the stove. The wicks will burn down until they light the cardboard on fire. The cardboard acts as a secondary wick, increasing the light and heat given off by the stove.

To use this for cooking, place a pot support 6 to 8 inches over the flame. Ensure that there are holes in the pot support to allow oxygen to get to the single-use stove. A 3-pound coffee can works for a pot support. You'll need to cut holes in the top and bottom to allow the free flow of oxygen to feed the flame.

🐝 Pinecone Fire Starters

Pinecone fire starters make lovely gifts. They are a fragrant way to get the fire going on cold winter mornings. This project is another good use for waste wax and bits of wick trimmed off from other projects.

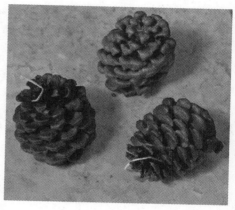

When you replace your powdered baking spices, use the old spices for this recipe. Dried and powdered orange peel or other citrus peels give a wonderful scent, as well. For gift giving, package 10 or 12 pinecones in a tin or brass pail to be kept beside the fire place. They'll scent the room with their honey-sweet holiday scent.

MATERIALS

12 to 20 ponderosa, lodgepole, or long needle pinecones

4 yards #2 or larger wick

3 cups melted waste beeswax

¼ cup powdered cinnamon

¼ cup dried, powdered orange peel

EQUIPMENT

Newspaper

Parchment paper

DIRECTIONS

1. Prepare the pinecones by soaking them overnight in cold water to remove any bugs or debris. Lay them out on newspaper and allow them to dry completely.

2. Prepare one wick that is at least 6 inches long for each pine cone. Spiral the wick around the pine cone from the widest part at the stem end of the pine cone to the narrowest part at the pointed end. Leave one-half inch of the wick hanging out at the pointed end. This will be the top of your fire starter.

3. Create a double boiler using a deep wax pot. Melt the beeswax over medium heat. The can should be wide enough to accept the pinecones without any obstruction. Stir in the powdered cinnamon and orange peel and mix thoroughly.

4. Spread out parchment paper to hold the pinecones between dips in the hot wax.

5. Dip the first pinecone into the wax. Hold it there for 30 seconds. Lift it out slowly, just as if you were dipping a candle. Allow the wax to drip back into the pot until the dripping stops. The spices have a tendency to sink to the bottom of the pot, so stir them into the wax as you are dipping.

6. Lay the pinecone on the parchment paper to cool. Repeat with all the pine cones.

7. Dip the pinecones a second time, using the same method as you did the first time.

8. Allow to the pinecones to cool. If desired, dip a third time to fully coat the pinecones.

9. The pinecones should harden for at least 48 hours before using.

TO USE

The pine cones are aromatic and can be placed in a basket near the fireplace to scent the room air until they are needed to light a fire. To use, light a fire in the fireplace or wood stove. Place kindling on top of the logs. Place a pinecone on top of the kindling. Light the wick on the pinecone fire starter. As the wick catches the wax on fire, the pinecone will burn as a secondary wick. The kindling will catch fire, which will light the logs on fire. Once the kindling is on fire, add dry wood on top of the burning kindling to increase the flame.

🐝 Solid Fuel Fire Starter

This fire starter uses up waste from around the house, as well as waste wax from the wax melting pot. They aren't pretty, but they are useful. Use this on those damp, cold, snowy winter days when there is no draw in the chimney; when you're camping, the weather is drizzly and miserable, and you're having trouble getting the fire going; or at the cottage after a day of cross country skiing.

I didn't give proportions for this recipe because you can use what you have and fill in the details. Have lots of waste wax? Fill a dozen muffin cups. Have only a bit of waste wax? Just make one or two for emergency fire starters. You'll be glad to have them on hand when you need them.

MATERIALS

Cardboard egg cartons

Cardboard toilet paper tubes

Dryer lint

Shredded paper

Bits of hemp or cotton string

¼ cup waste wax for each fire starter

Bits of wax crayons

Waste wicks left from trimming candles

EQUIPMENT

Silicone muffin pan

Baking sheet

Bobby pins

1. Place the silicone muffin pan on a baking sheet for support. Separate the individual egg cups from a cardboard egg carton. Place one egg cup in each silicone muffin cup. Cut cardboard toilet paper tubes in half. Place one half in each cardboard egg cup.

2. Fill the cardboard tubes with dryer lint, shredded paper, and bits of hemp or string. Pack the tube loosely to allow for the wax.

3. Place the waste wax and bits of wax crayon in a tin can, inside a double boiler. Simmer the wax until it melts.

4. Work the wicks down inside the tubes of scraps, leaving about one-half inch exposed at the tops. Secure these with bobby pins to keep them in the center of the tube.

5. Pour the wax into each tube, letting it fill the egg cup. Allow the wax to cool. Add additional wax to top up the tube.

TO USE

Light the wick and paper shreds to start a fire. Add kindling and dry wood to maintain a fire.

Leather Care

Leather needs the conditioning, cleaning, and waterproofing that beeswax formulas can offer. Commercial leather cleaning and dressing products contain silicone, polymers, and petroleum products that prevent leather from absorbing water. They also prevent leather from absorbing oils that would keep the hide soft and supple. Over time these can cause the leather to become brittle and dried out.

The following should not be used on artifact or collectible leather pieces. Instead, follow conservators' best practices with all artifact and collectible leather. These recipes are intended for sports and leisure uses of leather, where the leather is intended for regular use.

✳ Saddle Cleaning

Cleaning leather is the first step to reconditioning it. Beeswax soap removes old wax and oil, petroleum products, silicone dressings, and plastics from the leather; unclogs the pores; and prepares leather to absorb the leather dressing.

INGREDIENTS

Basic Beeswax Soap (page 106)

TO USE

1. Brush off any mud or dirt with a dry brush.

2. Using a sponge that is barely damp, work up some suds with the beeswax soap. When a thick, creamy lather is obtained, wash off every part of the leather by rubbing it with the dry lather. If there are belts or straps, draw them through the suds. Wipe off with a rinsed but wrung-out sponge to remove the last bit of dirt.

3. Use as little water as possible. The leather should be only slightly damp. Once every part of the piece has been cleaned with the soap, the leather needs to be conditioned.

4. The dampness allows the leather to absorb the leather dressing more efficiently. While the saddle is still damp, apply Leather Dressing (page 213).

✳ Leather Dressing

Dressing leather is the second step in conditioning leather, after cleaning. The objective is to replace the natural oils that were originally in the living hide, while providing a moisture barrier to keep the hide pliable and soft. This recipe contains natural animal fats to condition the hide. From boots to saddles and even baseball mitts, beeswax is a natural alternative to synthesized leather conditioners.

Applying a leather dressing will darken leather. Test in an inconspicuous spot before committing to doing the entire leather piece.

YIELD: 1 (5-ounce) container

INGREDIENTS

2 tablespoons beeswax

1 teaspoon carnauba wax

1 teaspoon pine resin

3 tablespoons tallow

5 tablespoons lanolin

DIRECTIONS

1. Create a double boiler using a glass jar. Simmer beeswax, carnauba wax, pine resin, tallow, and lanolin in the jar over medium heat to melt the wax. Stir together. Remove from the heat.

2. Continue stirring while the mixture cools.

TO USE

1. Apply with a light hand on both the grain side and the flesh side of freshly cleaned, still scantily damp leather using a soft cloth or your fingers. Rub it in evenly. Allow the mixture to dry for twenty-four hours out of direct sunlight.

2. Use a towel reserved for this purpose to polish the leather on both sides in a circular motion and with a good amount of elbow grease. This removes any unabsorbed oil and distributes the oil evenly through the hide.

3. Apply regularly to keep leather supple.

🌿 Leather Boot/Cowboy Boot Balm

This paste wax is easy to apply with a soft cloth to your shoes and boots, protecting them from moisture.

YIELD: 1 (4-ounce) tin

INGREDIENTS

2 tablespoons beeswax

2 tablespoons avocado butter

1 tablespoon tallow

2 tablespoons lanolin

DIRECTIONS

1. Create a double boiler using a glass jar. Simmer beeswax, avocado butter, tallow, and lanolin in the jar over medium heat to melt the wax. Stir together. Remove from the heat.

2. Continue stirring while the mixture cools.

3. Pour into a tin.

TO USE

1. Apply to clean leather using a soft cloth or your fingers. Use a light hand on the grain side. Rub it in evenly. Allow this to dry for 30 minutes.

2. Buff the leather to remove excess leather butter.

3. Repeat regularly to keep leather supple.

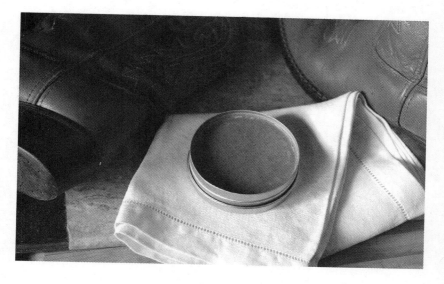

🐝 Shoe and Boot Polish

While other leather conditioners are meant to deeply penetrate leather goods, adding protection and suppleness, shoe polish is a surface coat that improves the looks and adds some waterproofing to leather shoes and boots. Commercial shoe polishes are made with polymers, naphtha, turpentine, petroleum distillates, and dyes, none of which are natural leather conditioners. They are both toxic and flammable. This natural, nontoxic shoe and boot polish can be made in a few minutes and is a superior product that will increase the life of your boots and shoes.

You can customize the color to match your shoes using oxide powders. The powders should be ground finer, using a coffee grinder, before use. Use a grinder with a removable stainless steel cup to make clean up easier. Grinding oxide pigments can also be done in a stone mortar and pestle.

YIELD: 1 (4-ounce) tin

INGREDIENTS

2 tablespoons beeswax

1 teaspoon carnauba wax

2 tablespoons cocoa butter

3 tablespoons walnut oil

1½ teaspoons brown or black oxide powder (optional, to customize the color)

DIRECTIONS

1. Create a double boiler using a tin can. Simmer beeswax, carnauba wax, cocoa butter, and walnut oil in the can until the beeswax and cocoa butter are melted. Stir together.

2. If using, micronize the oxide powder in a coffee grinder or with a mortar and pestle to make it very fine. Wear a mask to protect your lungs.

3. Remove a small portion of the melted wax mixture to a separate dish. If using, stir the micronized oxide powder into the wax, making a smooth paste. Return this colored wax mixture to the tin can and stir well to incorporate.

4. Pour the mixture, while warm, into a tin.

TO USE

1. Rub onto leather in a circular motion, making a thin, even coat. Allow to dry for 30 minutes.

2. Buff to remove excess polish and increase shine.

🐝 Dubbin

The word "dub" means to dress leather. Dubbin is used to condition and waterproof leather boots, drum skins, and other leather gear. It is meant to be rubbed thoroughly into the leather. Leather should be warmed before use to allow the dubbin to penetrate it more easily.

YIELD: 2 (2-ounce) tins

INGREDIENTS

1 tablespoon beeswax

2 teaspoons pine rosin

4 tablespoons tallow

1 tablespoon lanolin

¼ teaspoon cod liver oil

¼ teaspoon pine essential oil

DIRECTIONS

1. Make a double boiler using a glass measuring cup. Melt together the beeswax, pine rosin, tallow, and lanolin in the double boiler. Stir the mixture well to fully incorporate the pine rosin.

2. Stir in the cod liver oil. (Warning: This can smell pretty awful. I use lemon-flavored cod liver oil.) Remove from the heat.

3. Stir as the mixture cools to prevent the beeswax from clumping. When the mixture is cool to the touch, stir in the pine essential oil.

4. Pour into tins.

TO USE

1. Brush leather off with a dry brush to remove dirt and debris. Warm the leather to room temperature. Apply a thin, even coat of dubbin with a soft cloth in a circular motion, allowing it to penetrate into the leather. Dry for 30 minutes to an hour.

2. Rub off the excess with a clean cloth.

Target Sports

These recipes are designed to save money, customize your products using the best ingredients for the purpose, and avoid toxic chemicals that can foul up your health. Your sport shouldn't make you sick.

✳ Archer's Bowstring Wax

Archer's wax protects the bow-string from wear and offers tackiness and grip for more accurate shooting.

YIELD: 3 (1-ounce) containers

INGREDIENTS

3 tablespoons beeswax

2–3 tablespoons pine resin (add up to 3 tablespoons for a stickier grip on the bow)

1 tablespoon lanolin

Push-up container

DIRECTIONS

1. Create a double boiler using a glass measuring cup. Melt beeswax, pine resin, and lanolin inside the measuring cup over medium heat, stirring to fully mix the pine resin.

2. Remove from heat. Stir while it cools to prevent it from clumping.

3. Pour into push-up containers for ease of use.

TO USE

Apply the archer's bow-string wax to a piece of scrap leather. Use the leather to apply it to the bow-string. The friction from the leather helps the wax adhere to the bow-string.

Black Powder Shooting Lubricant

Shooting black powder pistols requires a grease lubricant to soften the carbon residue left by the black powder. When the barrel is without lubrication, the inside of the gun barrel gets hard, rough carbon deposits, which foul up the gun chamber and inhibit the smooth trajectory of the ball. The shooting lubricant, when used regularly, softens this carbon deposit and keeps the barrel smooth so that every shot can be accurate. Use less beeswax in winter for a softer lubricant.

The lubricant should be cleaned from the gun barrel at the end of the day.

YIELD: 5 (1-ounce) containers

INGREDIENTS

2 tablespoons beeswax

8 tablespoons tallow

¼ teaspoon sweet orange essential oil (optional)

DIRECTIONS

1. Create a double boiler using a tin can. Melt the beeswax and tallow in the can over medium heat. When the mixture is liquid, remove from the heat. Stir while the mixture cools.

2. When it is cool enough that you can place your hand on the side of the can without being burned, add the sweet orange essential oil, if using.

3. Pour the mixture into push-up tube containers.

TO USE

Take a lentil-size piece of lubricant and rub it on one side of the felt pad that separates the black powder from the slug. Place the felt pad so that the greased side faces the slug. Load as usual.

☀ Bore Butter

Bore butter is used to lubricate the bore of the gun in black powder shooting, reducing friction and increasing accuracy. It is used in the same way as the black powder shooting lubricant recipe above to prevent fouling the gun chamber with a hard carbon deposit. Petroleum-based lubricants should never be used in black powder guns due to the risk of hard fouling, which can ruin the barrel of the gun. Instead, edible grease and beeswax are used to keep the barrel clean and the carbon deposits soft.

This is not a rust preventative. The bore butter should not be placed in the powder chamber. The powder must remain dry.

YIELD: 1 (3-ounce) container

INGREDIENTS

2 tablespoons beeswax

4 tablespoons olive oil

¼ teaspoon peppermint essential oil

DIRECTIONS

1. Create a double boiler using a tin can. Melt the beeswax and olive oil in the can over medium heat. When the mixture is liquid, remove from the heat. Stir while the mixture cools.

2. When it is cool enough that you can place your hand on the side of the can without being burned, add the peppermint essential oil.

3. Pour the mixture into a push-up tube container.

TO USE

Take a lentil-size piece of the lubricant and rub it on one side of the felt pad that separates the black powder from the slug. Place the felt pad so that the greased side faces the slug. Load as usual.

✳ Bullet Lube

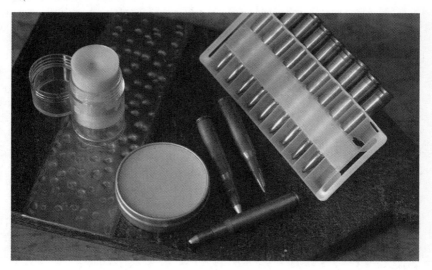

For those who reload their bullets, bullet lube ensures a cleaner barrel. The bullet lube is applied with the fingers to the ridges on the bullet before it is placed in its casing.

Bullet lube reduces friction and ensures that the first shots of the day are just as accurate as the last shots of the day. Bullet lube should be formulated to the ambient temperatures and humidity in your location. In colder climates, a less solid lube is preferred; use less beeswax in relationship to other oils. In warmer areas, use more beeswax in the ratio.

The carnauba wax in this formula helps to keep the barrel cleaner.

YIELD: 3 (1-ounce) containers

INGREDIENTS

2 tablespoons beeswax

1 tablespoon carnauba wax

2 tablespoons tallow

1 tablespoon lanolin

1 tablespoon castor oil

DIRECTIONS

1. Create a double boiler using a tin can. Melt the beeswax, carnauba wax, tallow, and lanolin in the can. Stir together to fully melt.

2. When the mixture is liquid, remove from the heat. Stir in castor oil. Continue stirring while the mixture cools.

3. Pour the mixture into push-up tube containers for ease of use.

TO USE

Take a lentil-size piece of the lubricant and rub it in the grooves of the bullet before it is placed in its casing. Load as usual.

Active Sports

Whether your game is rock climbing, golf, skiing, or surfing, beeswax can improve your day with superior grip, a smoother ride, and better recovery. These beeswax recipes can replace the cheap, petroleum-based ingredients and chemicals that commercial products rely on. With beeswax, after a day on the mountain or in the surf, you'll only leave behind memories, not residual toxins that will live for centuries in the environment.

🐝 Rock Climber's Hand Balm

The dry chalk of the rock face combined with jagged sharp rocks and blistering rope burns make rock climbing a painful, if exhilarating, sport. It's not unusual to see bloody fingerprints on the rock walls at the climbing gym. Clearly, if you are a climber, you need this balm. Honey and beeswax are humectant, moisturizing, and protective. Calendula and lavender promote skin health. Tea tree, lavender, calendula, honey, and beeswax are antimicrobial.

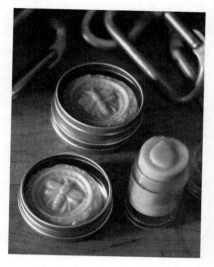

Many rock climbers prefer a solid lotion bar rather than a paste-like balm for ease of application. Use a mold for this bar that fits inside a tin container, and tuck one in with your climbing gear. To make the calendula-infused olive oil, use one of the methods of making an herb-infused oil on page 62.

YIELD: 3 (1-ounce) tins

INGREDIENTS

2 tablespoons beeswax

2 tablespoons cocoa butter

2 tablespoons calendula-infused olive oil

1 teaspoon honey

15 drops lavender essential oil

15 drops tea tree essential oil

DIRECTIONS

1. Create a double boiler using a glass measuring cup. Heat beeswax, cocoa butter, and infused oil in the measuring cup over medium heat until the beeswax is fully melted. Remove the

glass measuring cup from the saucepan and the saucepan from the heat.

2. Add honey to the beeswax mixture and stir well to fully incorporate.

3. Add the essential oils. Stir while the mixture cools so that the beeswax doesn't clump.

4. Prepare molds by applying silicone release spray, if necessary. When the mixture is still warm to the touch, pour it into the molds.

5. Let the hand balm firm up for several hours before unmolding. Wrap individually in paper and place in tin containers. Label.

TO USE

Rub the bar through hands, rolling it around between your palms and fingers to get adequate coverage. This will feel greasy at first but will be quickly absorbed within 5 or 10 minutes.

Baseball Glove Conditioner

Hand-me-down gloves need a little TLC to get them into top shape. Brand new gloves need breaking in to make them pliable and responsive. Some players swear by canned shaving cream, a product that contains silicone and will injure the leather over time. This glove conditioner contains lanolin, a natural leather preservative and softener.

Some players use liquid oils to soften and condition leather. But liquid oils can make the glove heavy and slick. Solid oils and lanolin condition the leather without weighing it down or making it slippery.

Use of this product will darken leather, so test it first in an inconspicuous spot.

YIELD: 1 (4-ounce) tin

INGREDIENTS

2 tablespoons beeswax

2 tablespoons cocoa butter

2 tablespoons avocado oil

2 tablespoons lanolin

DIRECTIONS

1. Create a double boiler using a glass measuring cup. Melt beeswax, cocoa butter, avocado oil, and lanolin in the glass cup over medium heat.

2. Stir well to incorporate.

3. Pour into a 4-ounce tin.

TO USE

Warm the glove by placing it in the sun or in a warm part of your home. Wipe the leather conditioner on the outside of the glove using a cloth and rub in using a circular motion. When the conditioning is done, place a ball in the palm of the glove to hold the shape while the glove conditioner dries.

Buff the glove to remove excess glove conditioner.

Golf Club Grip Wax

For barehanded golfers, grip wax takes away the slick and gives you more control over your game.

YIELD: 1 (2-ounce) container

INGREDIENTS

3 tablespoons beeswax

1 tablespoon powdered pine resin

DIRECTIONS

1. Create a double boiler using a tin can. Melt together the beeswax and pine resin over medium heat. Stir well to incorporate. Remove from the heat.

2. Stir as mixture cools to keep the pine resin incorporated with the beeswax. When it begins to thicken, pour into a push-up container.

TO USE

Rub your hands over the top of the grip wax as needed to provide grip.

How Beeswax Can Help You Better Your Golf Gear

Golfing requires a big investment in gear. Protect your investment with these beeswax products that you can make at home. You'll make a higher quality product than you can buy in the store, and you'll save money, too.

Golf wood conditioner. If you have antique woods, clean and condition them with Tool Handle Preservative on page 184.

Golf club shaft preservative. Prevent rust on the chrome shafts of your clubs by using one of the metal preservatives in Chapter 6.

Golf bag leather conditioner. Use the Leather Dressing on page 213 to clean and condition your leather golf bag.

Clean and condition your golf shoes. Brush the cleats with a dry brush to remove any dirt. Use the Shoe and Boot Polish recipe on page 216, but omit the mineral color. Titanium dioxide can be added to spiff up white shoes.

Snowboard and Ski Glide Wax

Common ski and snowboard waxes contain perfluorocarbon compounds, like Teflon, that are dangerous to the environment as well as damaging to the health of those applying the wax. The wax doesn't stay on the bottom of the skis with use. With every run, small amounts of waxing compound drop onto the snow pack and into the environment. These compounds are also extremely toxic when heated and cause health problems in the ski shop. There are very few organic waxes available that minimize the environmental impact of the sport.

Wax reduces the friction between the snowboard and the snow surface. It makes sliding easier by adding lubricity. It prevents ice crystals from sticking to the base of the skis or board, and keeps the base well hydrated to prevent damage. Glide wax can be customized to give better control in different snow conditions. Racers may need to tweak the following recipe for their snow conditions.

Beeswax is a durable wax that is a good binder. In warm, wet conditions, it provides increased speeds; however, it is gummy and hard to scrape during hot wax application. Adding other, harder waxes to beeswax improves the performance of the wax while maintaining its natural, eco-friendly composition.

The following recipe is an all-weather glide wax, which performs best in temperatures above 10°F. In the warm, wet snow conditions

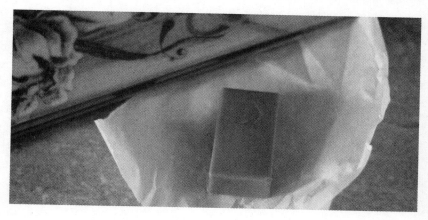

of early spring, increase the jojoba oil in the mixture to 1 tablespoon and omit the carnauba wax. In extreme cold, increase the carnauba wax to 1 tablespoon and omit the jojoba oil.

Powdered graphite is often added to ski wax to reduce static. Only a pinch is necessary to improve glide in extreme weather conditions.

YIELD: 1 (4-ounce) bar

INGREDIENTS

3 tablespoons beeswax

2 teaspoons carnauba wax

6 tablespoons candelilla wax

2 teaspoons jojoba oil

2 teaspoons orange wax

⅛ teaspoon powdered graphite (optional)

DIRECTIONS

1. Create a double boiler using a tin can. Melt together the beeswax, carnauba wax, candelilla wax, jojoba oil, and orange wax over medium heat. Stir together well. Once all the waxes are melted, remove from heat.

2. Stir the mixture while it cools. When it cools to a paste-like consistency, stir in the powdered graphite, if you are using it. Blend well.

3. Pour into a 4-ounce bar mold. Allow the bar to cool overnight. Wait 48 hours for the crystalline structure of the wax to reestablish before using.

TO USE

Clean and tune the bottom of a board or ski. Apply the wax using a hot iron reserved for ski waxing procedures. Apply the wax to the plate of the iron using the lowest temperature that will allow the wax to drip on the surface of the board or ski. Drip the melted wax over the surface of the bottom of the ski or snowboard. When the surface of the ski is covered in melted wax, use the iron at the lowest temperature to spread the warm, liquid wax over the full surface of the ski or board. Always use the lowest heat that will melt the wax. Allow the wax to cool, set, and penetrate the bottom of your ski overnight. Don't rush this.

Remove excess wax using a scraper. Brush the base from tip to tail using a variety of brushes, progressing from coarse nylon to soft horse hair. You want to leave a fine, even layer of wax over the surface of the ski or snowboard. Finally, buff the waxed bottom of the ski to produce a shine.

🦟 Surfboard Wax Bar

Board wax allows the surfer to grip the board without falling off when the board surface is slick from the water. Board wax is formulated according to the water temperatures in the area where the surfer rides.

Two wax coats are applied the board. The first wax coat leaves a pebbly surface, reducing slip, while the second wax coat offers some stickiness. In warm water, beeswax creates grip; in colder water, the addition of pine resin creates grip.

Make one board wax bar with pine resin to use as the base coat for the surfboard wax. If you are surfing in warm water, make a second bar of wax, omitting the pine resin for the top coat.

Base Coat
YIELD: 1 (4-ounce) bar

INGREDIENTS

4 tablespoons beeswax

1 tablespoon coconut oil

1 tablespoon pine resin

2 tablespoons calcium carbonate

1 teaspoon titanium dioxide

DIRECTIONS

1. Create a double boiler using a tin can. Melt the beeswax and coconut oil in the can over medium heat. When the beeswax is fully melted, stir in the pine resin. Continue stirring until the pine resin is fully melted. When the mixture is liquid, remove from the heat.

2. Stir while the mixture cools. When it is cool enough that you can place your hand on the side of the can without being burned, stir in the calcium carbonate and titanium dioxide.

3. Use a whisk to mix the calcium carbonate and titanium dioxide so that they don't clump. Continue stirring with the whisk until the mixture has the consistency of a soft paste and is just warm to the touch.

4. Pour the mixture into a silicone bar mold. Allow to harden for at least 24 hours before using.

Top Coat

YIELD: 1 (4-ounce) bar

INGREDIENTS

4 tablespoons beeswax

1 tablespoon coconut oil

1 tablespoon pine resin (optional)

DIRECTIONS

1. Create a double boiler using a tin can. Melt the beeswax and coconut oil in the can over medium heat. When the beeswax is fully melted, stir in the pine resin, if using. Continue stirring until the pine resin is fully melted. When the mixture is liquid, remove from the heat.

2. Stir while the mixture cools.

3. Pour the mixture into a silicone bar mold. Allow to harden for at least 24 hours before using.

TO USE

Remove old surfboard wax with a wax comb before applying fresh wax. Lay down a base coat of wax by rubbing the bar of wax in long strokes rail to rail on the board, covering the area of the board where your feet grip, plus 6 inches on either side. Lay down a second coat of wax moving the bar from tip to tail, covering the same area as in the first application. Finally, lay down a third coat of wax, moving the bar in a crisscross pattern across the same area. The wax will leave a pebbly surface to reduce slipping and give better grip. Wait 8 to 12 hours after applying the base coat before applying the top coat.

Apply the top coat according to the temperature of the water you will be surfing in. Use a cold water wax, with pine resin, for water temperatures below 70°F. Use the top coat recipe without the pine resin for warmer water temperatures. Apply the top coat by brushing the side of the wax bar in long strokes on the board. Apply a second coat. Allow to harden before using.

Chapter 9

BEESWAX AND THE ARTS

The artists must be sacrificed to their art. Like the bees,
they must put their lives into the sting they give.

—Ralph Waldo Emerson

Wax is such an integral part of every facet of life that it shouldn't be any surprise to find it is also an important assistant in the arts. Musical instruments are held together and lubricated with beeswax. While beeswax and resins provide protective varnishes, the sound of stringed instruments is made melodious with the help of beeswax, too.

Fiber artists have used beeswax as well to pattern cloth, while visual artists use beeswax as a paint binder, model maker, and medium.

Children's art materials are also made with beeswax and include modeling compounds, crayons, pastels, and paint.

Important documents and love letters have been sealed in beeswax. Beeswax is such an integral part of human cultural expression that some say that good will triumph over evil only if beeswax continues to be used in art.

Natural Dyes and Mineral Pigments

Many of the natural ingredients in this chapter are the same ingredients you used previously to create personal care products, build your apothecary, preserve and protect your home and garden, and play in the great outdoors. Beeswax along with these other natural ingredients figure largely in art mediums, modeling compounds, and even music.

You may have noticed as you read the recipes in this chapter that pigment and beeswax are used together in many of the art projects. If you're taking the time to make your own art supplies, it's definitely worth it to use natural colors and earth pigments. (If you want to delve into more details on pigments and natural dyes, see Resources on page 278.)

Natural vegetable-based colors are unpredictable, but that is part of their attraction. Mineral pigments, oxides, and ultramarines are more predictable and uniform. Soil pigments can also be found where you live, although you won't know their chemical composition. You may even design your own local palette as the artists of history did.

Red—red oxide mineral pigment, Australian red clay, alkanet root, carmine, and alizarin lake pigments

Pink—beet root powder (very pale), rose hip extract (very pale), hibiscus powder, titanium dioxide plus red oxide pigment, cochineal bugs with titanium dioxide

Orange—annatto (bright orange), alkanet root plus turmeric (burnt orange), yellow oxide plus red oxide

Yellow—turmeric (gold), yellow oxide mineral pigment, yellow ocher soil

Green—spirulina algae powder, chlorella algae powder, green oxide mineral pigment, French green clay

Blue—ultramarine blue mineral pigment, natural indigo powder, natural woad powder

Purple—purple ultramarine mineral pigment

Brown—red ocher soil, brown ocher soil, brown oxide, cocoa powder, coffee powder, black walnut powder, burnt umber mineral pigment, alkanet root

Black—charcoal, black oxide powder

White—titanium dioxide

Titanium dioxide is added to other pigments in small amounts to make them more opaque, which makes the color seem richer. In large amounts, titanium dioxide will make a pastel shade with the pigment. Black is added to other pigments, in small amounts, to darken or sadden (dull) the shade. A wide variety of shades can be achieved with a single-colored pigment and varying percentages of titanium white or one of the black pigments.

Red, blue, and purple pigments are the hardest to achieve using natural colors. Vegetable red colors can shift with pH changes, whereas mineral reds often lean toward brown. Cochineal bugs offer a strong red pigment in water-based applications, but in oil-based applications,

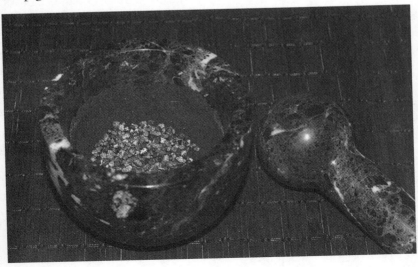

the rich carmine color is elusive. Cochineal pink is reliable when mixed with titanium dioxide. A stronger red can be achieved by making a lake color and then utilizing the resulting precipitated pigment, as opposed to using the ground bugs. Blues can be obtained from natural indigo or woad. But without a reliable red, the purple shades are hard to achieve using natural dye colors. Ultramarine purple is a synthetic color that is considered nontoxic.

Powdered natural dyes can be found at natural dye suppliers. You can even extract your own dye pigments from garden plants. It requires time and patience, but it's not expensive. Pigment extraction is an interesting science project for homeschoolers. (See Resources on page 278.)

When using mineral pigments like oxides, ultramarines, micas, or lake pigments, a little goes a long way. One teaspoon of pigment is enough for most of these recipes. However, when using some vegetable-sourced colors you'll need to experiment to get the depth of color you want. Indigo, carmine from cochineal bugs, and alizarin from madder are very strong colors. One-half teaspoon may be enough to give you a very rich shade of color in a crayon or pastel. Try 2 teaspoons of alkanet root (brown), annatto, (bright orange) turmeric (gold), spirulina (green), or chlorella (green). Use 2 tablespoons of cocoa, coffee, or black walnut powder for a deep rich brown.

Mixing the pigment with oil before combining it with your beeswax recipe will help the pigment stay suspended in your wax as it cools.

One more thing: vegetable-based colors have a definite odor that you don't find in chemical colors. Indigo, for instance, is made by fermentation, and there is a definite *odor d'compost* when mixing it as a pigment. You can mask this with essential oils. It isn't so obvious in the finished wax crayon, but it's there. Turmeric has its distinct fragrance, too. Consider yourself warned.

Wearing a dust mask, grind the pigment finely as you would to make mineral makeup. You can grind it in a coffee grinder reserved for pigments or with a mortar and pestle. Mix the measured pigment with a scant amount of the oil-based binder, blending from the edges to the center with a palette knife until the right consistency is achieved.

Make up a few tablespoons at once and you'll have them on hand for all the recipes in this section of the book.

Natural Indigo Dyeing

At our farm, workshop participants are always excited when I teach about natural indigo dyeing. The craft involves traditional dye-resist techniques like shibori, ikat, or batik to decorate silk scarves or cotton quilting fabric.

Batik uses wax as a resist to prevent areas of the fabric from being dyed when the fabric goes into the dye vat. Since wax melts easily at high temperatures, the dye must be able to adhere to the fabric without the use of heat.

Indigo *(Indigofera tinctoria)* was the traditional dye used with these techniques because it is a vat dye that dyes in barely warm water and doesn't require heat to set the color. Indigo can be grown in your backyard if you live in a place with a warm climate and a long growing season. The fresh plant material is used for dyeing. Alternatively, powdered indigo can be purchased and used for this project. In colder climates, woad *(Isatis tinctoria, I. indigotica)* can be used in place of indigo (see Resources on page 278). Indigo gives you varying shades of blue to purple natural color. The color depth depends on the length of time that the cloth remains in the dye vat, as well as the number of times the cloth is dipped. The final color on dry cloth will be paler than the perceived color as the cloth comes out of the dye bath.

Modern dyers often use fiber-reactive dyes with batik. Fiber-reactive dyes are synthetic dyes that form a chemical bond with cotton, linen, and hemp fibers in cold water. Precautions must be taken when using these dyes because the dyes are toxic in their powdered, unreacted form. Fiber-reactive dyes are available in every color. Follow the manufacturer's instructions for their use and take all necessary precautions to protect your health.

Traditionally, beeswax was used in batik because it is a soft wax that gives a clean, uncrackled appearance in the final piece. Many dyers today prefer the crackled look that paraffin wax gives to batik. Paraffin wax is brittle and tends to crack and peel off the fabric, leaving areas unprotected from the dye. Microcrystalline wax is often used to give the crackled look without flaking off.

🐝 Batik with Natural Indigo Dye

If, like me, you prefer a smooth, uncrackled look in batik, use 100 percent beeswax in your designs. If you prefer the crackled look, use a 50/50 blend of beeswax and paraffin or microcrystalline wax in the following project.

Whether you decide to use silk, cotton, linen, or rayon for this project, the method is the same. Silk needs a gentler hand when removing the wax in the final step. High heat can damage the luster of silk.

You will need a tjanting tool, the metal tool that keeps the wax hot long enough to draw your design on the fabric, for this project.

MATERIALS

1 silk scarf or 15 inches by 15 inches 100% natural fabric made of linen, cotton, or rayon

6 tablespoons beeswax (or 3 tablespoons beeswax and 3 tablespoons paraffin wax)

Batik/tjanting tool

Stencils (optional)

DIRECTIONS

1. Several hours before you plan to make your batik, prewash the fabric to remove the sizing. Dry the fabric and press any wrinkles.

2. Two hours before you plan to make your batik, prepare the indigo dye vat. (See The Magical Indigo Vat, page 239.)

3. Prepare a double boiler using a glass measuring cup. Melt the wax in the cup over medium heat.

4. Apply the wax to define your design using a tjanting tool. Ensure that the wax soaks through to the back of the fabric rather than remaining on the surface. Apply additional wax if necessary to fully cover the design. Allow the wax to harden on the fabric. Repeat with more fabric. You'll want to have several textiles ready for the indigo vat. Allow for at least an hour for the wax to fully harden.

5. Immerse your design in the indigo vat for five minutes. Remove the fabric from the indigo vat and allow it to oxidize 5 minutes. This oxidization is the magical part of the process. The fabric emerges from the dye bath a lime green color and over the next few minutes, it will transform to a deep blue shade as the dye molecules oxidize on the surface of the fabric. The dye color will build up with subsequent dips in the dye bath until shades of dark navy blue are achieved. Repeat the dye process as many times as necessary to achieve a deep shade of blue. The color will appear darker when wet.

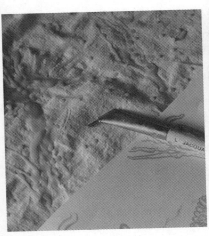 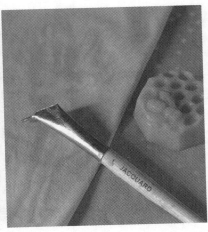

6. After the fabric has oxidized sufficiently, rinse the article in a pail in barely warm water. Change the water and rinse again until the rinse water runs clean. In the final rinse, add 1 tablespoon of white vinegar to the rinse water to buffer the higher pH of the indigo vat.

7. Hang the fabric to dry. Allow it to dry fully before removing the wax.

🐝 The Magical Indigo Vat

Natural indigo is a pigment that needs to reduce in a dye vat in order to adhere to fabric as a natural dye. A chemical reaction at a high pH must take place to turn the blue indigo to leucoindigo, a colorless indigo that gives the dye vat a chartreuse color. When properly reduced, a blue indigo scum will form on the top of the indigo vat where it encounters oxygen. The liquid under the scum will remain greenish.

Cloth immersed in the vat will appear to take on the green color of the vat. However, when the cloth is removed from the vat and exposed to air, the green transforms into blue right before your eyes. The magic comes from a chemical reaction whereby the indigo molecule gives up an oxygen atom. When the cloth comes out of the vat and is exposed to oxygen, those hungry indigo molecules grab the oxygen molecules that they need and the cloth is transformed.

There are many ways to reduce the indigo in the vat. Bacterial fermentation will reduce the vat overnight. This can be achieved with additions to the vat like sweet fruit, dates, or henna. See Resources on page 278 for information on creating an organic fruit reduction vat. Alternatively, the vat can be reduced by chemical means using the following recipe. Wear gloves and protective clothing when working with natural dyes.

YIELD: 9 quarts, enough to dye ½ pound of cotton fabric or 1 pound of silk fabric a dark blue shade

INGREDIENTS

Stock Solution

2 tablespoons natural indigo

1 teaspoon thiourea dioxide

2 teaspoons washing soda

3½ cups hot (140°F) water

Dye Vat

2 gallons hot (140°F) water

1 teaspoon washing soda

1 teaspoon thiourea dioxide

DIRECTIONS

1. **Stock solution:** Add the indigo, thiourea dioxide, and washing soda to a wide-mouth mason jar. Add the hot water and stir well to get rid of any lumps. Loosely cover the jar and let it sit for one hour. The surface of the jar will gain a coppery sheen with blue bubbles. The jar will take on a brownish color as the indigo is reduced.

2. **Dye vat:** Prepare a dye vat by filling a large pot three quarters full with hot water. Add an additional 1 teaspoon of washing soda and 1 teaspoon of thiourea dioxide to remove oxygen from the water. When the stock solution is ready, lower the jar into the pot and pour it out under the surface of the water to avoid adding oxygen to the water. Stir gently and cover. Allow the vat to reduce another 30 minutes.

3. The dye vat is ready when the dye solution is lime green and there is coppery blue sheen on the surface of the vat.

Wax Removal

4. Fully immerse the cloth in a pot of hot water. You may need to weigh the cloth down to keep it submerged. It must stay below the surface of the water so that the wax doesn't re-attach to the fabric. Bring the temperature to 160°F to fully melt the beeswax. Silk can be damaged at temperatures over 185°F, so watch the

temperature of the water carefully if you are using silk. Cotton and other vegetable fibers can handle more heat than silk. Turn off the heat. Leave the cloth submerged in the water until the water returns to room temperature. Don't pull the cloth out of the pot through the wax; skim the wax off the surface of the water first. The wax may be reused.

5. Remove the cloth from the pot. Don't dump the water with the wax down the drain. Residual wax can harm indoor plumbing.

6. Wash the cloth in soap and water and line dry. Press to remove wrinkles. Admire your art.

✳ Sealing Wax

Sealing wax must adhere to paper or parchment, which is flexible. It must be flexible enough not to peel off or break when handled, yet it must be brittle enough to break when the document is opened so that it can't be reaffixed, proving the document has not be tampered with. Finally, it must melt in a flame and shrink when cold, so as to take a clean impression of a wax stamp. This is a tall order. Beeswax alone doesn't make a good seal because it is too flexible. It can easily be peeled off and reaffixed.

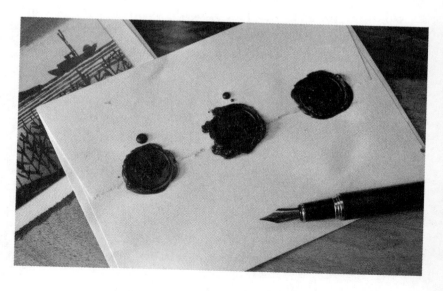

For this recipe, prepare molds using tin foil to make the classic sealing wax–shaped bullet, or use a silicone crayon mold. You may want to spray the mold with mold release to make it easier to use.

YIELD: 4 (1-ounce) molds

INGREDIENTS

4 tablespoons pine resin

1 tablespoon gum turpentine

2 tablespoons beeswax

1 tablespoon prepared natural dye pigment (see **Natural Dyes and Mineral Pigments, page 233**)

15 drops peppermint essential oil (optional)

DIRECTIONS

1. Create a double boiler using a tin can. Simmer the pine resin in the tin can on medium heat until the resin begins to melt. Once the pine resin is melted, stir in the gum turpentine and beeswax. Stir until the beeswax is fully melted. Remove from the heat.

2. Add the prepared natural dye pigment to the beeswax mixture. Stir well to fully mix the dye pigment with the wax mixture.

3. Continue stirring while the mixture cools slightly. Add the essential oil, if you wish. When the mixture begins to thicken, pour into prepared molds.

4. Allow the mixture to harden in the molds overnight. Wait 48 hours to use.

TO USE

Prepare your seal impression by lightly coating the metal seal with water. If you have a lot of seals to make, leave your seal on a damp sponge between uses.

Warm the tip of the sealing wax stick in a candle flame just until a blob of sealing wax begins to form on the end of the crayon. Twirl the stick in the flame to encourage even melting of the crayon.

Place the blob of sealing wax over the seal of an envelope to create a circle of wax slightly bigger than the diameter of your seal. Press firmly with your metal seal. Lift off cleanly. Allow the wax to harden.

Note that wax-sealed envelopes should be placed inside another plain envelope to be sent through the mail.

Beeswax is a natural nonhazardous material for creating **art supplies**. Beeswax has longevity. Combined with quality pigments, artwork made from beeswax has been known to last for centuries. But it's not just for Van Gogh. Children's art supplies can be made with beeswax and colored with food stuffs or nontoxic pigments, offering an alternative to the standard paraffin, petrolatum-based products in the school supply aisle.

While you can use gel food coloring or melted crayons to color your own art supplies, it's only a little extra effort to use natural colors and earth pigments see Natural Dyes and Mineral Pigments on page 233.

Beeswax Crayons

Every fall, boxes of crayons come home with the school supplies. Most crayons are made with paraffin wax and stearic acid. Soy crayons are made with hydrogenated genetically modified soy bean oil. Some brands of crayons may contain lead and asbestos. So while technically, crayons are "nontoxic," they are not necessarily benign.

You could make crayons by melting beeswax and adding a pigment. The resulting crayons are softer than commercial crayons and don't perform well. Adding carnauba wax and cocoa butter to this recipe results in a harder crayon that performs well. Choose your pigment from natural vegetable pigments, earth pigments, or gel food colorings.

YIELD: 5 (1-ounce) crayons

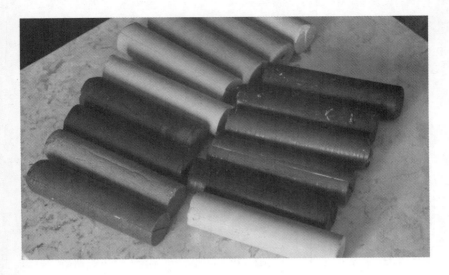

INGREDIENTS

Silicone mold

¾ cup beeswax

2 tablespoons cocoa butter

6 tablespoons carnauba wax

1 teaspoon each of 5 different natural pigments (see Natural Dyes and Mineral Pigments on page 233)

DIRECTIONS

1. Make a double boiler using a glass measuring cup. Simmer beeswax, cocoa butter, and carnauba wax in the cup over medium heat until the beeswax is melted.

2. Prepare five different pigments while the beeswax is melting.

3. Remove the wax mixture from the heat. Divide the wax base into five portions of one-fourth cup each.

4. Working with one portion at a time, return the remaining portions to the hot water bath to keep them melted. Stir the prepared pigment into one portion, being careful to suspend it fully in the wax. Use a clean spatula for each pigment.

5. Continue stirring while the mixture cools slightly, to prevent the pigment from settling to the bottom of the mixture. When the mixture begins to thicken, pour into your prepared crayon molds.

6. Repeat with each additional crayon color.

7. Allow the crayons to harden for several hours until they are cool to the touch.

🐝 Beeswax Pastels

YIELD: 2 (1-ounce) pastels

INGREDIENTS

2 tablespoons white beeswax

2 tablespoons jojoba oil

2 teaspoons prepared oil–based pigments (page 278) or natural pigments (page 233) for each color

DIRECTIONS

1. Create a double boiler using a tin can. Bend a pouring spout on the can with a pair of pliers. Simmer the beeswax and jojoba oil in the can over medium heat until the beeswax is melted. Remove from the heat.

2. Stir in the pigment, evenly distributing it with the pigment in the wax mixture. Continue stirring while the mixture begins to cool.

3. Pour mixture into prepared molds.

4. Allow the pastels to harden fully before removing from the mold. They will be ready to use in 24 hours.

5. Repeat this recipe for each color you require.

Oil-Based Pigments

Some beeswax recipes call for color to be added in the form of crayons. Crayons already have oil-based pigments added. However, such crayons may have petroleum-based waxes that you don't want to add to your organic art supplies.

These oil paints are made using a drying oil (like walnut oil, raw flaxseed oil, or safflower oil), beeswax, and pigment. It's a two-part process to make your own oil-based pigments using oxides, mineral pigments, or micas, the same ones you used to make mineral makeup in Chapter 3. Other powdered natural dye pigments can also be used to make oil-based pigments.

🌿 Making an Oil Medium and Pigment

First, you'll need to make a small amount of oil medium that combines a drying oil with beeswax. The second step is to add color to the oil medium, which is absorbed by the pigment and carries the grains of the pigment. An oil medium also helps you grind the pigment more finely, if you wish, using a mortar and pestle or a glass plate and a muller. Once you have the oil-based pigment, you can use it in any of these beeswax art supply recipes as a coloring agent, instead of dyes or melted crayons.

Each pigment is different in how it behaves in the oil medium. Ultramarine blue may require a higher percentage of beeswax in the oil medium to make a uniform paste.

INGREDIENTS

½ cup walnut oil

1 teaspoon white beeswax

Variety of oxide, mica pigments, or powdered natural dye colors

EQUIPMENT

Glass palette

Palette knife

Glass dropper

DIRECTIONS

1. Make a double boiler using a glass measuring cup. Simmer the walnut oil and beeswax mixture in the cup just until the beeswax melts. Stir this thoroughly. Remove from the heat.

2. Allow mixture to cool naturally, stirring occasionally to achieve a uniform mixture. Pour into a small jar with a tight fitting lid.

3. Wearing a dust mask, place 1 teaspoon of pigment on a glass palette. Make a hollow in the middle of the pile with your palette knife. Drop oil medium from the glass dropper into the hollow, beginning with just a few drops.

4. Stir the oil medium into the pigment, drawing the pigment at the edge of the pile into the center with the palette knife. Continue adding a small amount of the oil medium and mixing the pigment into the oil medium until all the pigment has been moistened by the oil medium and the mixture has a smooth, uniform consistency.

5. If the particles of pigment are clumpy or gritty, use a muller or pestle to press them firmly into the oil medium, reducing the particle size and encouraging more oil to be absorbed by the pigment.

6. Continue to work the pigment from the outside to the center of the pile with the palette knife until you have a smooth, even consistency.

7. The pigment should mound up and hold its shape, with the consistency of toothpaste or cake fondant. If it's too liquid, add more pigment. If it's too dry, add more oil medium, a few drops at a time. When the pigment has a smooth, thickened consistency, it is ready to use in any of the recipes in this section.

8. You can also use this pigment to paint an oil painting, as is. Unused pigment can be stored in a paint tube or small jar for later use.

✳ Beeswax Modeling Clay

Beeswax modeling clay is a tactile and sensory art material commonly used in Montessori and Waldorf education programs. Homeschoolers also use beeswax clay. Beeswax clay is unique because the colors can be separated out after use and returned to their color families for storage. Beeswax clay has a long shelf life. Purchasing beeswax clay can be pricey, but you can make your own using natural beeswax.

You can use wax crayons to tint this modeling clay. Most wax crayons are made from petroleum products. You can also add oil-based pigments that you make yourself.

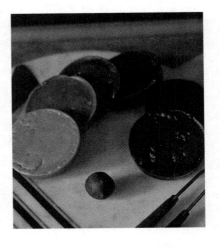

YIELD: 6 discs

INGREDIENTS

½ teaspoon plus 5 teaspoons jojoba oil

1 cup beeswax

2 teaspoons lanolin

6 wax crayon colors or 6 teaspoons natural oil-based pigments

Silicone mold

DIRECTIONS

1. Rub the inside of a glass measuring cup with ½ teaspoon of jojoba oil to make it easier to clean. Create a double boiler with the glass measuring cup. Simmer the remaining jojoba oil, beeswax, and lanolin in the cup over medium heat until the beeswax is fully melted. Divide the beeswax into 6 portions of 2 tablespoons each.

2. If you are using wax crayons for pigments, add one-fourth of a wax crayon for color into each portion. You'll need a full crayon for white. Pour the beeswax mixture into prepared

silicone molds. The crayon won't be melted at this point. Place the silicone molds into the oven at 200°F. Allow the crayons to melt. Remove from the oven and stir the beeswax to fully blend the color into the wax.

3. If you are using oil-based pigments for the color, prepare them from oxide and mica colors (page 66). Stir 1 teaspoon of oil-based pigment into each portion. If the color is not intense enough, you can add more pigment. There is no need to put the beeswax in the oven if you are not using crayons for the pigment.

4. Allow the beeswax modeling clay to cool completely in the molds. The clay is ready to use after it's hardened.

TO USE

Soften the beeswax in your hands or place in a glass of warm water. The clay will not dry out and can be used over and over.

Beeswax Oil-Based Clay (Plasticine)

Plasticine was invented in 1897 by British art teacher William Harbutt. He wanted non-drying clay that could be used over and over for his students. The original formula is top secret, but it was made with a blend of petrolatum, gypsum, and paraffin wax.

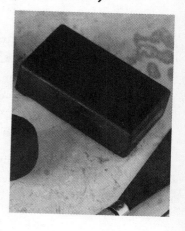

The clay is used extensively in children's art classes. It is used in animation because it stays pliable and doesn't melt or dry out under studio lights. Sculptors use oil-based clay to create models to use for mold casting. Bomb squads, military, and medical personnel also use it.

YIELD: 3 bars

INGREDIENTS

6 tablespoons beeswax

2 tablespoons lanolin

2 tablespoons jojoba oil

2 tablespoons cocoa butter or 1 tablespoon stearic acid

¾ cup calcium carbonate

3 tubs gel food coloring or 1 tablespoon natural oil-based pigment for each color. (Use only 1 teaspoon of natural indigo, if using.)

DIRECTIONS

1. Prepare silicone molds for the bars. Make a double boiler using a tin can. Simmer beeswax, lanolin, jojoba oil, and cocoa butter in the can over medium heat until the beeswax and cocoa butter are melted. Remove from the heat.

2. Slowly stir in the calcium carbonate. Stir well to make sure that there are no clumps. Continue stirring until the mixture forms a stiff dough and all the calcium carbonate has been added.

3. Test the consistency of the mixture. It should be soft and pliable and hold its shape when pinched or rolled. If it shears apart or crumbles when you try to mold it, return it to the can, re-melt it, and add more cocoa butter or beeswax. If it is too slippery, add more calcium carbonate. If it feels too firm, add more jojoba oil, 1 teaspoon at a time.

4. Divide the mixture into three equal portions. Stir a separate pigment color into each portion. Press the colored oil-based clay into silicone molds to set overnight or for at least 12 hours.

TO USE

Use as a modeling clay. Colors can be blended by rolling and kneading two primary colors together. Clay will not dry out.

Mixed Media Collage

Mixed media collage is a creative technique that uses layers of paint, found materials, wax, and resins to create art. The technique is usually applied to abstract art. Pinterest is full of inspiration for mixed media collage. Consider adding beeswax to your collage.

If you feel intimidated, begin with a small canvas. Use a block of wood or an artist trading card for your foundation canvas. It doesn't have to be large.

Gather found materials like pieces of lace, newspaper, or magazine pictures. The collage is built in layers beginning with a foundation layer of paper and paint.

On the second layer, add cut-out pictures, pieces of lace, cut-out words from newsprint, stickers, and found items.

A layer of melted wax can be added and textured with or without pigment. This is an opportunity for creative expression.

Add pigment to the wax or use natural wax, spread it smooth with a palette knife, or texture it and build up layers.

Continue until you have a pleasing effect. In the final layer, use beeswax as a light coating of varnish to ensure that your work endures.

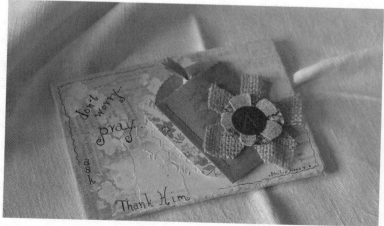

This small mixed media collage was a gift from my friend, artist Sandy Kaye Moss of Ohio. Sandy used a small canvas panel as a base for her collage.

Encaustic Painting

My neighbor Vivien is an encaustic artist. She brings her supplies to artisan shows and sits at her table with a hot iron, dripping and daubing melted wax pigments on paper. Lately she's been making cards with her art. There is a definite fragrance to her work, of beeswax candles and paint. My own encaustic art looks more like melted crayons on canvas compared to Vivien's expert hand.

Encaustic painting uses a white filtered beeswax and resin medium, combined with pigments. The medium is applied to boards, canvas, pottery, or paper, either as a cold cream wax, which is applied with a palette knife at room temperature, or by melting the medium with a hot iron. The softened wax medium is then used for drawing or painting. Cold cream wax can be manipulated at room temperature like oil paint. Wax that is applied hot can be manipulated and textured before it cools. The wax can also be reheated and reworked for different effects. The result is a textured, brilliantly colored painting that will maintain its integrity and luminosity for centuries.

Pliny the Elder described the encaustic technique in the first century. It was used by the Egyptians in their sepulcher art. Later, icon painters made use of it in church art. In the 1990s, there was a revival of interest in encaustic painting. See Resources on page 278 to find out more.

❋ Encaustic Medium for Hot Wax Techniques

This wax medium will hold your natural pigments so that you can use them with encaustic painting techniques or with mixed media collage. The addition of damar resin gives shine to the work.

YIELD: 1 (4-ounce) block

INGREDIENTS

1 tablespoon damar resin crystals

½ cup beeswax

1 to 3 teaspoons prepared pigment

DIRECTIONS

1. Make a double boiler using a tin can. Melt the damar resin in the can over medium heat. Damar resin crystals melt at 225°F. You may need to put your melting tin directly on the bottom of the double boiler rather than on a ring to get them to melt.

2. Once the resin is melted, stir the beeswax into the melted resin to fully combine. The resin tends to settle on the bottom of the container, so you'll need to scrape it from the bottom and stir it into the wax several times. If you have difficulty combining the resin with the beeswax, place the tin can directly on the surface of an electric frying pan to increase the heat enough to fully melt the resin crystals.

3. Once the mixture is fully incorporated, stir in the prepared pigment. Remove from the heat.

4. Continue to stir the mixture with a spatula while the mixture cools. When it begins to thicken like honey, pour into a block mold. Allow this to harden completely. After 48 hours, it's ready to use with your encaustic technique or with mixed medium collage.

5. Repeat this procedure for each color of encaustic block you want.

Beeswax has many uses in music. One of the most ancient uses is in the maintenance of the bagpipe. A bar of pure beeswax is used to coat the hemp thread used on bagpipe tuning slides and tenon joints. The hemped joint handles the wet-dry cycles of instrument-playing well, as the beeswax prevents the hemp from absorbing too much moisture while being played, as well as preventing shrinkage during dry periods, which would cause the joint to loosen.

My husband's dad played the bagpipes, and my husband and I both play the clarinet. Originally, the tenon joints on woodwind instruments were covered in hemp thread that was waxed with beeswax.

Bagpipes continue to be hemped today. Other woodwind instruments now have cork on the tenon joints. The cork doesn't handle the wet-dry cycle as well as waxed hemp did.

Wind players go through a fair bit of cork grease to keep those corks soft and resilient. My vivid memory of high school band was the rancid smell of the cork grease tin. Even new cork grease had that "off" smell.

Modern cork grease is made from petroleum products like paraffin wax and petrolatum. Over time, this clogs the pores of cork, reducing

Pysanka

Pysanka, or Ukrainian Easter eggs, are meticulously decorated eggs. The word "*pysanka*" comes from the root word "*pysaty*," meaning "to write," because the traditional designs are not painted on the egg, but instead, written with beeswax. The beeswax acts as a resist, much like in batik. Areas that are waxed repel the dye. Several dye colors are used and the wax is blotted off and reapplied in different areas between dye baths. The layering of dye colors leaves a black or dark brown overall color to the egg, while the design shows through in brighter colors. The result is luminous. Sometimes only a few dye colors are used, resulting in a lighter, brighter egg.

Other Slavic cultures also make these beautifully decorated eggs. The traditional motifs are passed down through family lines and have highly symbolic meanings. Even the colors used represent life, happiness, hope, and rebirth. One egg may take as much as 11 hours to complete. In a typical household, as many as 60 eggs are decorated in late winter by the women to be given to family and friends at Easter.

The decorated and dyed eggs predate Christianity in Slavic culture. They were important parts of sun god worship, symbolizing the rebirth of the earth in spring and used in fertility rites and as protective talisman.

There is a myth that the making of pysanka is essential to the continuation of the world. If at any time the custom of decorating eggs ceases, evil and chaos will overrun the world.

the wood's ability to absorb moisture, compress, and rebound. This leads to the disintegration of the cork structure and a loosening of the glue on the tenon joint of the instrument. The loose tenon joint lets air leak, which spoils the tone of the instrument and results in expensive repairs.

Cork Grease

Making beeswax cork grease is as simple as making lip balm. Try this recipe that uses beeswax and lanolin, two ingredients in traditional cork grease. Natural beeswax cork grease won't harm the cork or the glue. The lanolin in this mixture will replenish the oils in poorly maintained corks, adding lubrication and improving the fit in the tenon joint. It won't go rancid like that old tin of Rico cork grease in your instrument case. And you can use this on your lips, too, as some players do, without ingesting petroleum by-products.

YIELD: 1 (2-ounce) container

INGREDIENTS

1 tablespoon beeswax

2 teaspoons lanolin

1 tablespoon cocoa butter

1 tablespoon coconut oil

10 drops peppermint essential oil

DIRECTIONS

1. Make a double boiler with a glass measuring cup. Simmer the beeswax, lanolin, cocoa butter, and coconut oil in the cup over medium heat until the beeswax and cocoa butter melt. Mix well. Add peppermint essential oil.

2. Pour into lip balm sticks or a push-up tube for ease of application. Allow the mixture to cool completely before using.

Violin Rosin

Violin, cello, and bass rosin is one of the best-kept secrets of the luthier trade. The recipe has been kept a closely guarded secret for centuries. Violin rosin is made from blends of beeswax and conifer resin, with other ingredients that modify the stickiness or bite of the bow on the strings. It is the stickiness of the bow across the strings that vibrates the string and gives voice to the instrument.

Softer, dark rosin is used in colder weather and for deeper instruments like bass and cello. Lighter, harder rosin is used for violas and violins, the higher-voiced instruments. Modifiers can be added to the rosin to make it harder or softer, or to modify the friction of the bow. Additives like powdered gold, silver, and copper are added to modulate the grip on the string and therefore the sound of the instrument. Violin rosin is mostly pine or larch resin, the same plant product that is used in sports to increase grip. Beeswax is added to make it more stable and a little less sticky to handle.

Since pine resin is a natural product, the quality of the resin varies during the growing season and from year to year.

YIELD: 1 (4-ounce) bar

INGREDIENTS

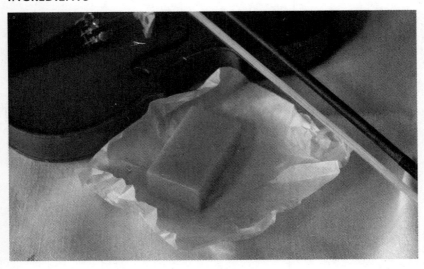

DIRECTIONS

1. Prepare a heavy mold that can withstand high heat. Use mold release spray. The ingredients are extremely hot. Avoid burns.

2. Make a double boiler using a tin can. Pine resin is sticky. Don't use your best pots for this one.

3. Place pine resin in the tin can and simmer over medium heat until the pine resin becomes liquid. Stir with a disposable wooden stick to encourage the process. Rosin manufacturers do this over direct heat, which is faster than the double boiler.

4. Add beeswax and carnauba wax as soon as the resin becomes clear, and continue stirring to melt the wax. Once the mixture is fully liquid, pour into the prepared mold. Allow to set for several hours, until the rosin is solid and cold to the touch. It will be better to wait 48 hours before using, to allow the crystalline structure of the rosin to reestablish after melting.

5. Use this as you would any violin, viola, cello, or bass rosin. Keep good notes. Since each instrument has a different need for grip on the string and each player has their personal preference, you can tweak this recipe for your specific need. If you need a softer rosin, replace the carnauba wax with more beeswax. If you need a harder rosin, replace a portion of the beeswax with carnauba wax. Add gold dust or fairy dust to get the violin rosin you prefer. And then feel free to join the age-old tradition and keep your special recipe a secret. Enjoy the freedom of making your own rosin.

Chapter 10

INGREDIENT GUIDE

The sage gathers wisdom as the bee gathers honey.

—Proverb

With a well-stocked supply cupboard, you'll be able to make all the projects in this book. You'll get the best results if you follow the recipes carefully, exactly as written, but I know that's not always possible. When ingredients are sourced internationally, there can be supply problems. Some of the rarer ingredients may be unavailable or out of your price range. You may be allergic to one of the ingredients and need a substitution.

I wanted the recipes in this book to be accessible to most people. I used a lot of different ingredients because I wanted you to become familiar with their attributes, freely making substitutions in a knowledgeable way to get the exact results you are looking for in each recipe.

Here you'll learn the rationale for choosing each ingredient and what you can substitute for that ingredient if you can't find it, you're allergic to it, or you run out. For some of the ingredients, there is no comparable substitute. I'll let you know if that's the case.

This might be more than you want to know. If so, you can skip this section. The recipes are formulated to work perfectly as they are. All the recipes will work just fine even if you don't know why they work the way they do.

Making Substitutions

Substitutions should be made on a cup for cup, tablespoon for table-spoon basis, unless otherwise noted. Don't be afraid to experiment. You can always put your concoction back in the double boiler and add more liquid oil, beeswax, or vegetable butter to get it to the consistency that you are looking for. Beeswax won't break down with reheating, provided you keep the temperature below 175°F. That's one of its miraculous attributes.

Keep in mind, though, that if you make substitutions, your product may not turn out exactly as planned. Keep good notes and don't be afraid to experiment through trial and error. You may come up with the perfect solution to a problem. With excellent notes, you can easily repeat your success.

Waxes and Emulsifiers

Beeswax

Shelf life: indefinite

All the recipes in this book were formulated specifically for use with beeswax, so don't try to substitute another wax. The recipes won't work with other waxes in the same way. However, you can substitute yel-low beeswax for white beeswax, and beeswax pastilles for solid beeswax. If the recipe calls for beeswax sheets, though, there is no substitute.

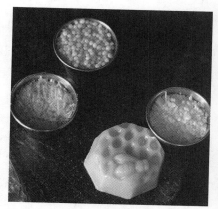

Clockwise, beginning at the top: candelilla wax, beeswax pastilles, rendered beeswax, carnauba wax.

Candelilla Wax

Shelf life: indefinite

Candelilla wax is extracted from the leaves of the wax slipper shrub (*Euphorbia cerifera*) using sulfuric acid. The wax is aromatic, hard, shiny, and brittle. Candelilla wax is used to harden other waxes without raising their melting point. It sometimes has a strong aroma that transfers through to the finished product.

Substitution: Candelilla wax is sometimes marketed as a vegan substitute for beeswax, although it lacks many qualities that beeswax has. You can substitute beeswax for candelilla wax; however, use twice as much beeswax as the candelilla wax called for in the recipe.

Carnauba Wax

Shelf life: indefinite

One of the hardest natural waxes, carnauba wax comes from the leaves of the palm *Copernicia prunifera*, grown only in Brazil; it's sometimes called "palm wax" or "Brazil wax." It's used in applications where its hardness and shine are of benefit. It is a common ingredient in shoe polish, surfboard wax, and leather and wood polishes to give shine and durability. It is often combined with beeswax. Used alone, it is brittle and tends to flake off the surface of objects. Carnauba wax is also used as a coating for pills and for candies, giving hardness and shine.

Carnauba wax melts at 187°F, a higher temperature than beeswax. In recipes, melt the carnauba wax first and then add the beeswax after the carnauba wax is liquid. This will protect the beeswax from breaking down in high temperatures.

Substitution: Carnauba wax has no substitute.

Jasmine Wax

Shelf life: 2 years if kept in a cool, dry place

Jasmine wax is a by-product of the extraction process of jasmine absolute perfume from jasmine blossoms (*Jasminum*). It has the strong scent of jasmine, as well as the therapeutic benefits of jasmine blossoms. Jasmine is an aphrodisiac, a relaxant, and helpful for menstrual pain. It is anti-inflammatory, antiseptic, adaptogenic, and can help balance energy levels and hormones. It can increase the milk supply in nursing mothers. It is used for its aroma in perfumes as a lingering bass note. It can be used in place of rose wax in perfumes. Jasmine softens the skin. It prevents scarring by increasing the skin's elasticity. It is expensive, but a tiny bit goes a long way.

Substitution: If jasmine wax is outside your budget, cocoa butter can be substituted. Without jasmine wax the product will not be exactly the same, but it will still be suitable.

Anhydrous Lanolin or Wool Wax

Shelf life: 1 year

Lanolin, the thick grease separated from the wool of merino sheep, is used as an emulsifier and moisturizer. It repels water and is protective of leather and wood products. It acts as a barrier to protect from harsh environments.

Traditionally, lanolin is added to leather care products to restore the natural oils to the leather that are removed during the tanning process. It is also used in shaving creams and soaps to moisturize and provide a barrier between the skin and the razor, protecting from nicks and scratches.

Substitution: You can substitute orange wax.

Orange Wax

Shelf life: 2 years

Orange wax is extracted from orange peels used in the food industry. The oil obtained is further processed to produce a dark colored, highly orange-scented, dark liquid wax. Orange wax is similar to the chemical structure of lanolin and is used in many recipes as a substitute for lanolin. It acts as a barrier in cosmetics. It has antimicrobial properties and is highly valued in wood care products, leather and wood conditioners, and polishes. Like orange essential oil, it can cause photosensitivity in susceptible people and should not be used in skin care products for people who are out in the sun all day. It is safe to use in nighttime skin care products, though.

I like to use it in kitchen wood care recipes because it has some cleaning power from the residual d-limonene left in the wax, as well as being protective and antimicrobial.

Substitution: If you choose to leave orange wax out, add sweet orange essential oil to the recipe—¼ teaspoon per ¼ cup of orange wax called for in the recipe.

Rose Wax

Shelf life: 2 years if kept in a cool, dry, place

Rose wax is a by-product of the extraction of rose absolute from Bulgarian rose petals (*Rosa* genus). It has an intense rose scent and contains the therapeutic, anti-inflammatory, anti-aging, astringent properties of roses. Used in small amounts in skin-care products and perfumes, it has antiaging properties and repairs and rejuvenates damaged skin.

Rose wax is expensive but a little bit goes a long way. One ounce of rose wax will make several recipes in this book. Rose wax can be omitted from the recipes if it is outside of your price range.

Substitution: Use mango butter or cocoa butter on a teaspoon-per-teaspoon basis. The finished product will not be exactly the same and it won't have the same benefits, but it will still be nice.

Borax

Shelf life: indefinite

Borax is essential for making lotions without the use of emulsifying wax. The recipes in this book use only a tiny amount of borax. If you decide to omit it, the recipe may not emulsify.

Substitution: Borax has no substitute.

Sunflower Lecithin

Shelf life: 9 to 12 months

Lecithin is fractionated from sunflower oil. It helps to emulsify oils and water to make lotions. Only a very small amount is used in these recipes. Beeswax is an incomplete emulsifier. The addition of borax and lecithin helps the formula to remain emulsified in storage.

Substitution: Sunflower lecithin has no substitute.

Butters

Vegetable butters add moisturizing and thickening properties to balms, lotions, and creams. In cosmetics and apothecary products, the butters are added for texturing and moisturizing. In this application they can be used interchangeably. In non-cosmetic products, they are added as a hardening agent or for a particular chemical fraction in their makeup.

Avocado Butter

Shelf life: 12 months

Avocado butter is a hydrogenated butter from the oil pressed from the avocado pit. Very soft at room temperature, it's especially useful for moisturizing older skin and repairing damaged skin. It is used in balms and ointments, as well as cosmetics.

Substitution: Mango butter can be substituted for avocado butter in skin care recipes on a tablespoon-by-tablespoon basis.

Cocoa Butter

Shelf life: 24 to 30 months

Creamy, rich cocoa butter is the fat of the cocoa bean *(Theobroma cacao),* the source of chocolate (the unrefined version smells of chocolate). At room temperature it has a waxy texture, but it melts at body temperature. It is a good addition to massage creams, lipsticks, and moisturizers, where it adds anti-oxidants, vitamin E, and a creamy texture. It gives hardness to soaps, crayons, and polishes because of stearic acid, which makes up one quarter to one third of its weight.

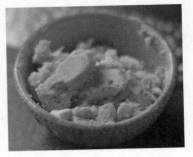

Substitution: In recipes where it is used for its stearic acid content, tallow or kokum butter can be substituted on a tablespoon-for-tablespoon basis. In cosmetic recipes, kokum butter is a good substitute.

Kokum Butter

Shelf life: 18 to 24 months

Kokum butter is pressed from the seed of the fruit of the mangosteen tree *(Garcinia indica)*. It is a hard, flaky oil used in cosmetics. It melts at body temperature. Kokum butter is 55 percent stearic acid.

Substitution: You can substitute cocoa butter on a tablespoon-for-tablespoon basis.

Mango Butter

Shelf life: 18 to 24 months

Mango butter is pressed from the seeds of the mango fruit *(Mangifera indica)*. It has a rich, creamy texture that is solid at room temperature but melts at body temperature. It adds richness and slip to cosmetic recipes. It is moisturizing and protective. It is used in antiaging products to soften the appearance of wrinkles and moisturize the skin.

Substitution: It can be used interchangeably for shea butter in cosmetic recipes.

Shea Butter

Shelf life: 12 to 16 months

Shea butter, from the nuts of the shea tree (Vitellaria paradoxa), is used to treat damaged, dry, weathered skin. It is naturally rich in vitamins A and E, as well as essential fatty acids. Avoid extreme temperature fluctuations and overheating when working with shea butter or it may become grainy. Shea butter offers low level sun protection (SPF 6) and helps with after-sun skin care. The unrefined butter has a strong aroma. Look for a refined version that is expeller-pressed and naturally deodorized, without the use of strong chemicals.

Substitution: Cocoa butter can be used in the place of shea butter on a tablespoon-by-tablespoon basis. The finished product will have a firmer texture. You can also substitute the more expensive mango butter.

Carrier Oils

Liquid at room temperature, carrier oils are so named because herbs can be infused in the oil for a short period. When the herbs are strained out, the beneficial portion of the herbs remains in the oil. The oil "carries" the benefit of the herbs into your cosmetics, balms, soaps, and ointments.

When infusing herbs into oil, I generally use olive oil as the carrier oil, unless I am looking for a specific quality in the oil I'm using. Olive oil is easy to find and inexpensive.

Other oils were used in these beeswax recipes not just to carry the benefits of herbs, but because they bring specific qualities to the final preparation. For instance, when using oils in a wood finish, wood conditioner, leather conditioner, or for waterproofing, it's important the oils dry relatively quickly rather than remaining in a liquid state. If you must substitute a carrier oil because of an allergy or a problem with availability, substitute a drying oil with another drying oil, or a non-drying oil with another non-drying oil.

Argan Oil

Shelf life: 18 to 24 months

Argan oil comes from the nuts of the argan tree *(Argania spinosa)* that grows in Morocco. It is a sought-after skin care and hair care oil that is one of the rarest oils in the world. It is rich in antioxidants, containing twice as much vitamin E as olive oil. It is a superior antiaging oil that softens the skin and removes the appearance of wrinkles by restoring the skin's water–lipid layer. It repairs the skin and helps to prevent stretch marks. It is very good for both hair and nails, and is used in after-shave products and hair conditioners.

Substitution: Argan oil is expensive. If this oil is outside your budget, sweet almond oil can be used instead. It won't have the same benefits but the finished product will still be nice.

Babassu Oil

Shelf life: 18 to 24 months

Babassu oil is extracted from the seeds of the fruit of the Babassu palm *(Attalea speciosa),* which is grown in South America. The oil is solid at room temperature but melts on skin contact. With similar properties to coconut oil, it is used in skin care, cleaners, and food.

Substitution: Can be used interchangeably with coconut oil.

Castor Oil

Shelf life: 24 to 36 months when kept in a cool, dry place

Castor oil, pressed from the seeds of the castor plant *(Ricinus communis),* is a heavy oil. You may have been given it as a laxative by the doctor, before x-rays. It is cathartic when taken internally. When used topically, it has many cosmetic uses. It adds shine to lip balms. It is valued in nail care, used to soften callouses and moisturize cuticles. It adds shine and volume to hair and increases the lather in shampoos and soaps when added in small amounts. When used in cold-processed soap, it can make the soap trace much faster than without it.

Substitution: Jojoba oil can be substituted for castor oil.

Coconut Oil

Shelf life: 18 to 24 months if kept in a cool, dry place

Coconut oil is pressed from fresh, mature coconuts *(Cocos nucifera)*. It is solid at room temperature but melts immediately upon contact with the skin. It absorbs into the skin at an average pace and leaves a light, oily feeling. Virgin coconut oil will have a light coconut scent.

Coconut oil is the preferred oil for direct use on the skin. It provides rich lather to soaps and creates a hard, drying bar of soap when used alone in soapmaking.

Substitution: For those who are allergic to coconut oil, babassu oil can be used in its place. When making substitutions in a soap recipe, please run your ingredients through a lye calculator to determine what adjustments need to be made in the lye fraction.

Raw Flaxseed Oil

Shelf life: 1 year in a cool, dry place, out of direct sunlight

Raw flaxseed oil is pressed from flaxseed *(Linum usitatissimum)*, grown for oil and linen fiber. The commercial product, boiled linseed oil, has heavy metals and toxic dryers. It should not be used in place of raw flaxseed oil in any of the beeswax recipes in this book. Raw flaxseed oil is the edible oil sold in grocery stores. It has useful emollients and is high in antioxidants and vitamin E. It is useful for helping with eczema and psoriasis. It is anti-inflammatory and beneficial for softening skin and easing scarring and stretch marks.

Flax is the number one drying oil. It can be heated in a double boiler over low heat to increase its drying qualities for use in waterproofing, wood care, and leather care.

Flaxseed oil may spontaneously combust due to the heat generated by the oil-soaked cloths. Cloth or paper towels soaked in flaxseed oil should be spread out on a rack to dry, to prevent combustion. Once the cloths are dry they are safe to store or discard.

Substitution: Hemp seed oil, grape seed oil, and walnut oil can be used in place of raw flaxseed oil on a cup-for-cup basis.

Grape Seed Oil

Shelf life: 2 years if kept in a cool, dry place

Grape seed oil is an odorless, light oil pressed from the seeds of grapes *(Vitis vinifera)*. It is a drying oil that is often used as a replacement for flaxseed oil for those who are allergic to flax or linseed. Grape seed is quickly absorbed by the skin and is used in cosmetics as a carrier oil. Massage therapists use grape seed oil because it doesn't leave a greasy feeling on the skin.

Substitution: Hemp seed oil, raw flaxseed oil, and walnut oil can be used in place of grape seed oil on a cup-for-cup basis.

Hemp Seed Oil

Shelf life: 1 year if kept refrigerated or in a cool, dry place

Hemp seed oil is extracted from the nut of the fiber hemp plant *(Cannabis sativa).* The oil is high in polyunsaturated fatty acids. It is anti-inflammatory, skin healing, and helps with joint pain. Hemp seed oil is a drying oil, used much like flax/raw linseed oil.

Substitution: Hemp seed oil can be used interchangeably with raw flaxseed oil, grape seed oil, or walnut oil on a cup for cup basis.

Jojoba Oil

Shelf life: 5 years

Jojoba is a liquid plant wax high in vitamin E and resists rancidity. It closely resembles the oil profile of human skin, making it an ideal carrier oil for moisturizers and ointments.

The jojoba shrub *(Simmondsia chinensis)* is native to Arizona, Southern California, and Mexico. During World War II, the oil was used as a lubricant in machine guns, motor oil, differential gear oil, and transmission oil. It was developed as a replacement for whale oil in cosmetics and for industrial uses. It is superior to whale oil in many uses.

It is an outstanding oil to use in skin and hair care products. It is also useful for leather care. Due to its high antioxidant levels, jojoba has a long shelf life.

Substitution: Jojoba oil has no substitute.

Olive Oil

Shelf life: 2 years if stored in a cool, dry space

Olive oil is pressed from the fruit pulp of the olive tree *(Olea euopaea)*. Most of the world's olive oil comes from the area around the Mediterranean, with some being grown in California. It is a favorite, all-purpose oil for both skin care and hair care. Olive oil is used extensively for herb-infused oils because it is a light oil with antioxidants and vitamin E, so it resists rancidity.

When a recipe calls for infused oil, infused olive oil may be used in place of the infused oil called for in the recipe.

Keep in mind that some olive oils found in North America have been adulterated with canola oil. Check your source of olive oil before using it in the recipes in this book. Canola oil is not a reasonable substitute for olive oil. Using adulterated olive oil in a soap recipe can affect the success of your final soap. Canola oil has a different saponification value than olive oil.

Substitution: Sweet almond oil, argan oil, or sunflower oil can be substituted in skin care recipes.

Pomegranate Oil

Shelf life: 2 years if kept in a cool, dry place

Pomegranate is one of my favorite oils for facial serums, moisturizers, and eye care. It is rich in antioxidants, soothing, and anti-inflammatory. Pomegranate oil comes from the dried seeds of the pomegranate

(Punica granatum). It is softening and nourishing to the skin. It has an average absorption rate and leaves the skin with a slight oily feeling.

I use it in tandem with rose hip seed oil and argan oil to stretch the more expensive oils in antiaging serums.

Substitution: Red raspberry seed oil, argan oil, or rosehip seed oil can be substituted successfully.

Red Raspberry Seed Oil

Shelf life: 2 years

Red raspberry seed oil *(Rubus ideaus)* is an antioxidant oil that is high in vitamin A. It has strong moisturizing and skin-healing qualities. Red raspberry seed oil contains an abundance of essential fatty acids: linoleic, alpha linoleic, oleic, omega-3, and omega-6. It has anti-inflammatory and skin-softening qualities. At full strength, red raspberry seed oil can act as a natural broad-spectrum UVA and UVB shield. It is a good oil for before-and-after sun care. It has a light raspberry fragrance. It is an expensive oil, best reserved for facial moisturizers and antiaging products.

Substitution: Red raspberry seed oil has no substitute.

Rose Hip Seed Oil

Shelf life: 6 months to a year

Rose hip seed oil is extracted from the seeds of roses *(Rosa genus)*. It is high in antioxidants and is a superior antiaging oil. It lessens the appearance of wrinkles, helps rebuild the skin, and heals scarring. It is useful for burns, including sun burn. It is an expensive oil and should be reserved for specialty skin creams and eye serums.

Rose hip seed oil is a drying oil. It is non-greasy and absorbs quickly. Rose hip seed oil should be stored in the fridge or in a cool location.

Substitution: Pomegranate oil can be substituted for rose hip seed oil, although the skin care qualities will be different.

Sea Buckthorn Oil

Shelf life: 2 years if stored in a cool, dark place

Sea buckthorn oil is pressed from the berries of the sea buckthorn shrub *(Hippophae rhamnoides)*. The oil is used in small amounts in facial moisturizers and antiaging products. In large amounts, it may stain the skin due to its deep orange color. The sea buckthorn berry contains the highest vegetable source of vitamin C, vitamin E, unsaturated fatty acids, and essential amino acids, along with beta-carotene, which makes the oil ideal for high-end skin care products. It should not be used as more than 10 percent of any skin care product to prevent the high beta carotene from staining the skin.

Substitution: Rosehip seed oil, pomegranate oil, or argan oil can be substituted for the small amount of sea buckthorn oil called for in a recipe. However, it is inadvisable to use sea buckthorn oil in the place of another skin care oil, due to the chance of staining the skin.

Sunflower Oil

Shelf life: 9 to 12 months

Sunflower oil is pressed from the seed kernels of the sunflower *(Helianthus annuus)*. It has high amounts of vitamins A, B, D and E, minerals, lecithin, insulin, and unsaturated fatty acids. It is an excellent skin care oil and helps heal sun-damaged skin. It absorbs into the skin at an average rate and leaves a light oily feeling.

Substitution: Sweet almond oil, argan oil, or olive oil may be substituted, but the skin care properties will differ.

Sweet Almond Oil

Shelf life: 2 years in a cool, dry place, out of direct sunlight

Sweet almond oil is pressed from the nuts of the sweet almond *(Prunus dulcis)*. The oil is light and nourishing, with very little fragrance. It is used extensively in skin care products. It softens skin and improves hair growth and hair health. It absorbs into the skin at an average rate and leaves a slight oily feeling.

Substitution: Olive oil can be used interchangeably with sweet almond oil in skin care recipes.

Tallow

Shelf life: 2 years at room temperature

Tallow is the rendered fat of sheep, goats, or cattle. It is a by-product of the meat industry. It is high in stearic acid and is used to harden some leather care products, soaps, and wood care products. It also provides lubrication for firearms. It is valuable because it doesn't go rancid at room temperature.

Substitution: Coconut oil, while emollient, doesn't contain high enough stearic acid fractions to be a suitable substitute. Instead, substitute cocoa butter or kokum butter in recipes where the stearic acid content is meaningful to the finished product.

Walnut Oil

Shelf life: 6 months to a year if kept refrigerated

Pressed from the kernels of Persian walnuts *(Juglans regia)*, walnut oil is used by artists and furniture makers because of its drying abilities. This drying oil is highly valued as a wood finish and preservative, especially on wood used in the kitchen. It is quickly absorbed by the skin and is useful for anti-aging products. It can be found in the grocery store in the salad oil section. Those who are allergic to tree nuts should substitute other drying oils for walnut oil.

Substitutions: Grape seed oil, hemp seed oil, or flaxseed oil can be substituted.

Essential Oils

Essential oils are highly concentrated extracts that carry the volatile oils of plants, flowers, and herbs, as well as their fragrance. Essential oils have therapeutic benefits, as well as antimicrobial, anti-inflammatory, and analgesic properties. In cosmetics, besides their therapeutic effect, essential oils offer flavor and fragrance to the final product.

When used therapeutically, the whole plant is of more benefit than the fractionated portion used in essential oils. Plants have synergy. Infused oils are used to provide the benefits of plants in the recipes in this book.

Essential oils vary greatly in their shelf life. Citrus oils are the most perishable, with a shelf life of 6 months to 1 year. Resinous essential oils like frankincense will keep for 2 to 5 years. The shelf life of essential oils can be prolonged if the oils are kept refrigerated and protected from light.

All essential oils should be stored out of the reach of children to avoid accidental poisoning.

Substitution: In many cases, the essential oil used in the recipes can be substituted for other essential oils that are less expensive, more pleasing, or more common. The final product won't have the same fragrance. Substitute drop for drop, unless otherwise stated.

Herbs

The herbs used in this book are infused in liquid oil and added in the oil portion of the recipe, unless otherwise noted. To make infused oil, see How to Make an Herb-Infused Oil (page 62).

The recipes in the cosmetic section of this book detail the quicker method of making herb-infused oil. In those recipes, previously prepared infused oils can be substituted for the quickly-prepared infused oils detailed in each recipe.

The shelf life of herbs varies greatly, with leaves and flowers lasting about 1 year and roots and fruit lasting 2 to 4 years. If an herb smells fragrant, it is still medicinally active. Herbs should be kept out of direct light and in a cool place for maximum shelf life.

HERB	Skin Healing	Cell Proliferant	Hemostatic/Styptic	Antimicrobial	Anti-inflammatory	Alterative	Nervine	Analgesic	Anti-fungal	Soothing
Calendula	x	x	x	x	x				x	x
Cayenne			x	x	x			x		
Chamomile				x	x			x		x
Comfrey	x	x	x		x					x
Dandelion	x			x	x			x		x
Eucalyptus				x				x		x
Garlic				x	x			x	x	
Ginger				x	x			x		
Lavender	x			x	x	x	x	x	x	x
Lemon balm				x	x					
Lemongrass				x	x				x	
Peppermint	x			x	x			x		x
Pine				x	x			x		
Plantain	x		x	x	x	x				x
Rose	x				x		x			x
Rosemary				x	x			x	x	
St. John's wort	x			x		x	x	x	x	x
Thyme				x	x			x		
Willow				x	x			x		
Yarrow	x		x	x	x		x	x		

Resins, Gums, and Solvents

Resins and gums add hardness, protection, and shine to the finished product. They are especially useful in wood care and leather care products where they act as a moisture barrier, as well as modifying the hardness of the final recipe.

Resins, gums, and solvents last indefinitely. Solvents should be protected from evaporation by being placed in a bottle and tightly capped.

All solvents should stored out of reach of children to avoid accidental poisoning.

Damar Resin

Damar resin is the hard gum resin from a tree in the West Indies. It is used to harden beeswax to raise its melting temperature for the encaustic art medium.

Substitution: There is no substitute for damar resin in encaustic painting.

Pine Resin

Pine resin is the gum from pine trees that has had the volatile oil of turpentine removed by heating. It is dry and hard. It is used to add stickiness and hardness to beeswax products. It melts at a higher temperature than beeswax. It should be melted first in the double boiler, with the beeswax added after the pine resin is melted to avoid damaging the beeswax with unnecessary high heat. It is used to enhance grip in sports products. It is the main ingredient in violin rosin.

Substitution: Other hard resins can be substituted for pine resin, such as spruce resin or larch resin.

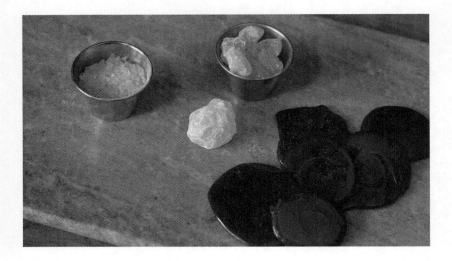

Gum Turpentine

Gum turpentine is the volatile oil distilled from raw pine sap, leaving behind pine resin. Gum turpentine is therapeutic and contains the pine fragrance. While industrial turpentine has added driers and petroleum distillates, gum turpentine should contain only the natural turpentine distilled from pine sap. Gum turpentine is especially useful for wood protection, wood finishes, and regular wood care.

Substitution: D-limonene is often used as a substitute for gum turpentine. However, d-limonene is a weaker solvent. For dissolving shellac or damar resin, gum turpentine should be used. Everclear may be used as a substitute for gum turpentine, especially when dissolving damar resin.

D-Limonene

D-limonene is a fractionated portion of the essential oil of sweet oranges. It has a strong orange fragrance. It is used in recipes as a solvent and cleaner. It is antimicrobial, yet safe for the skin. It won't burn the skin the way other solvents do. It is used as a hand cleaner and degreaser. When used in wood care, it cleans and protects without drying out the wood.

Substitution: Sweet orange essential oil can be substituted in some recipes where the d–limonene is not acting as a solvent. Where it is used as a solvent, gum turpentine is the better substitute, though you can use 80-proof vodka in a pinch.

99% Rubbing Alcohol

Rubbing alcohol is used as a solvent in some recipes because it is readily available. It is antimicrobial, but drying to the skin. It is a strong poison and must be kept out of the reach of children to avoid accidental poisoning.

Substitution: D–limonene, 80–proof vodka, or gum turpentine can be substituted.

Vodka

Vodka can be used in the place of other solvents in these recipes. Eighty-proof vodka can be used in the place of d–limonene or rubbing alcohol as a solvent. When used as such, the recipe will not be the same but it should have a similar texture.

RESOURCES

Many of the products used in the recipes in this book may be found locally at grocery stores. Those that can't be found locally can be ordered online. For more resources and to access how-tos and bonus content, see my webpage: JoybileeFarm.com/Resources-Beeswax-Workshop-Bonuses

Waxes, Oils, Butters, and Molds

Bramble Berry Soap Making Supplies
www.BrambleBerry.com
Ships from: Washington state

Bramble Berry has soapmaking supplies, lye (and an online lye calculator), molds, containers, mineral pigments, carrier oils, vegetable butters, essential oils, and beeswax.

FPI Sales North America
www.FPI-America.com
Ships from: Washington and Vancouver, Canada

This Canada-based company carries a good selection of essential oils, carrier oils, and body butters at wholesale prices and in large quantities.

Mountain Rose Herbs
www.MountainRoseHerbs.com
Ships from: Oregon

Mountain Rose Herbs sells organic herbs, carrier oils, vegetable butters, beeswax, and essential oils. They also carry a small selection of cosmetic containers. They have a large selection of organic medicinal herbs, as well as seeds to grow your own herbs.

New Directions Aromatics
www.NewDirectionsAromatics.ca
Ships from: Ontario, Canada

New Directions Aromatics sells soapmaking supplies, essential oils, mineral makeup supplies, carrier oils, and waxes, including orange wax, mineral pigments, and a small selection of containers at wholesale prices.

Saffire Blue
www.SaffireBlue.ca
Ships from: Ontario, Canada

Saffire Blue carries herbs, soapmaking supplies, molds, carrier oils, butters, essential oils, mineral pigments, beeswax, and other waxes, including floral wax.

Containers

SKS Bottle and Packaging
www.SKS-Bottle.com
Ships from: New York

You'll find a wide range of glass and tin containers suitable for every recipe at SKS Bottle and Packaging. Containers are sold in case lots at wholesale prices. Lids are sold separately. Shipping is fast.

Pine Resin and Gum Turpentine

Diamond G Forest Products
www.DiamondGForestproducts.com
Ships from: Georgia

This family-run business carries natural gum turpentine and pine resin from their own trees. While available on Amazon, it's less expensive to order directly from the company's website.

Natural Dyes, Pigments, and Batik Supplies

Maiwa

www.Maiwa.com

Ships from: Vancouver, Canada

Maiwa carries a variety of natural dyes, fabric, and batik supplies, as well as the tools for pysanka. Everything you need to dye with natural indigo, as well as detailed instructions, is available from their website. Maiwa's blog is a treasure trove of natural dye information.

Earth Pigments

www.EarthPigments.com

Ships from: Arizona

Earth Pigments offers mineral pigments, oxides, and ochers, as well as mullers and glass to grind your own pigments. They also carry damar resin. Full instructions are available on their website.

Dharma Trading Company

www.DharmaTrading.com

Ships from: California

Dharma's huge selection of ready-to-dye textiles includes silk scarves and fabric bolts. They also carry natural and synthetic dyes, tjanting tools for batik, and instructions for dyeing using beeswax resists.

Beeswax and Candlemaking Supplies

Busy Bee Candle Supply

www.BusyBeeCandleSupply.ca

Ships from: Ontario, Canada

Busy Bee Candle Supply carries molds and beeswax.

Wicks and Wax

www.WicksandWax.com

Ships from: British Columbia, Canada

Specializing in candlemaking, Wicks and Wax carries beeswax sheets, bulk beeswax, molds, and wicks.

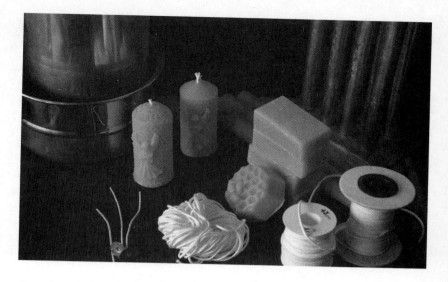

Beekeeping Supplies and Bees

Betterbee
www.Betterbee.com
Ships from: New York

Betterbee carries intricate silicone candle molds, wick, and beeswax. They have the reproduction tin molds for taper candles, as well as beekeeping supplies and kits for beginning beekeepers. They also carry packaging for selling your handmade candles.

Mann Lake
www.MannLakeLTD.com
Ships from: Minnesota

Mann Lake carries beekeeping and candlemaking supplies.

Urban Bee Supplies and Education
www.UrbanBeeSupplies.ca
Ships from: Vancouver, British Columbia

Urban Bee Supplies and Education carries beekeeping supplies, including queens, nucs (small honeybee colonies with a queen), and equipment.

Warré Beekeeping
www.Warre.Biobees.com
The company's website offers information on how to build a Warré hive.

Beekeeping Organizations

Canadian Honey Council
www.HoneyCouncil.ca

American Beekeeping Federation
www.ABFnet.org

Apimondia, International Federation of World Bee Keeping Federations
www.Apimondia.org

International Bee Research Association
www.Ibrabee.org.uk

Suggested Reading

Beeswax

Beeswax Alchemy: How to Make Your Own Soap, Candles, Balms, Creams, and Salves from the Hive by Petra Ahnert

Beeswax Crafting by Robert Berthold

Beeswax Crafts, Candlemaking, Modelling, Beauty Creams, Soaps and Polishes, Encaustic Art, Wax Crayons by David Constable, Polly Binder, and Norman Battershill

Candlemaking

The Candlemaker's Companion: A Complete Guide to Rolling, Pouring, Dipping, and Decorating Your Own Candles by Betty Oppenheimer

The Everything Candlemaking Book by Marie-Jeanne Abadie

Soapmaking

The Everything Soapmaking Book: Learn How to Make Soap at Home with Recipes, Techniques, and Step-by-Step Instructions by Alicia Grosso

The Natural Soap Book: Making Herbal and Vegetable-Based Soaps by Susan Cavitch

Pure Soapmaking: How to Create Nourishing, Natural Skin Care Soaps by Anne-Marie Faiola

Homemade Cosmetics

101 Easy Homemade Products for Your Skin, Health & Home: A Nerdy Farm Wife's All-Natural DIY Projects Using Commonly Found Herbs, Flowers & Other Plants by Jan Berry

Body Care Just for Men: Natural Health Tips & Herbal Formulas for Skin Protection, Sore Muscle Relief, Aftershaves, Tonics, and More by Jim Long

Make It Up: The Essential Guide to DIY Makeup and Skin Care by Marie Rayma

Herbs

American Household Botany: A History of Useful Plants, 1620–1900 by Judith Sumner

Homegrown Healing: From Seed to Apothecary by Christine Dalziel

Invasive Plant Medicine: The Ecological Benefits and Healing Abilities of Invasives by Timothy Lee Scott

Medicinal Plants of the Pacific West by Michael Moore

The Practice of Traditional Western Herbalism: Basic Doctrine, Energetics, and Classification by Matthew Wood

Rosemary Gladstar's Herbal Recipes for Vibrant Health: 175 Teas, Tonics, Oils, Salves, Tinctures, and Other Natural Remedies for the Entire Family by Rosemary Gladstar

Aromatherapy

The Beginners' Book of Essential Oils: Learning to Use Your First 10 Essential Oils with Confidence by Christine Dalziel

Carrier Oils: For Aromatherapy and Massage by Len Price and Shirley Price

The Complete Book of Essential Oils and Aromatherapy by Virginia Ann Worwood

Art and Music

Batik: 21 Beautiful Projects Using Simple Techniques by Diana Light

Earthen Pigments: Hand-Gathering & Using Natural Colors in Art by Sandy Webster

Encaustic Painting Techniques: The Whole Ball of Wax by Patricia Baldwin Seggebruch

Formulas for Painters by Robert Massey

The Organic Artist: Make Your Own Paint, Paper, Pigments, Prints, and More from Nature by Nick Neddo

Wax and Paper Workshop: Techniques for Combining Encaustic Paint and Handmade Paper by Michelle Belto

Beekeeping

Backyard Beekeeper by Kim Flottum

The Bee Friendly Garden by Kate Frey and Gretchen LeBuhn

Natural Bee Keeping: Organic Approaches to Modern Apiculture by Ross Conrad

Blogs and Websites

Attainable Sustainable
www.AttainableSustainable.net

Backyard Beekeeping Blog
www.BeeThinking.com/blogs/top-bar-hive-blog

Bad Beekeeping Blog
www.BadBeekeepingblog.com

Beekeeping like a Girl
www.BeekeepingLikeaGirl.com

Beverly Bees
www.BeverlyBees.com

Garden Therapy
www.GardenTherapy.ca

Humble Bee and Me
www.HumblebeeandMe.com

Joybilee Farm
www.JoybileeFarm.com (my website)

Maiwa
www.MaiwaHandprints.blogspot.ca

The Nerdy Farm Wife
www.TheNerdyFarmWife.com

Runamuk Acres Farm & Apiary
www.RunamukAcres.com

Schneider Peeps
www.SchneiderPeeps.com

Turning for Profit
www.TurningforProfit.com

Urban Overalls
www.UrbanOveralls.net

Wearing Woad
www.WearingWoad.com

BIBLIOGRAPHY

Al-Waili, N. S. "An alternative treatment for pityriasis versicolor, tinea cruris, tinea corporis and tinea faciei with topical application of honey, olive oil and beeswax mixture: an open pilot study." *Complementary Therapies in Medicine* 12, no. 1 (2004): 45–47. doi:10.1016/j.ctim.2004.01.002.

Al-Waili, N. S. "Clinical and mycological benefits of topical application of honey, olive oil and beeswax in diaper dermatitis." *Clinical Microbiology and Infection* 11, no. 2 (2005): 160–163. doi:10.1111/j.1469-0691.2004.01013.x.

Al-Waili, N. S. "Topical application of natural honey, beeswax and olive oil mixture for atopic dermatitis or psoriasis: partially controlled, single-blinded study." *Complementary Therapies in Medicine* 11, no. 4 (2003): 226–234. doi:10.1016/s0965-2299(03)00120-1.

Bridges, B. "Fragrance: emerging health and environmental concerns." *Flavor and Fragrance Journal* 17, no. 5 (2002): 361–371. doi:10.1002/ffj.1106

Glausiusz, Josie. "The Chemistry of . . . Mummies." *Discover Magazine,* March 1, 2002. Accessed June 13, 2016. http://discovermagazine.com/2002/mar/featchemistry

Henry, M., et al. "Reconciling laboratory and field assessments of neonicotinoid toxicity to honeybees." *Proceedings of the Royal Society B: Biological Sciences* 282, no. 1819 (2015). doi:10.1098/rspb.2015.2110.

Lewis, P. A., et al "A randomized controlled pilot study comparing aqueous cream with a beeswax and herbal oil cream in the provision of relief from postburn pruritis." *Journal of Burn Care & Research* 33, no. 4 (2012): 195–200. doi:10.1097/bcr.0b013e31825042e2.

Rezaei, K., Wang, T., and Johnson, L. "Combustion characteristics of candles made from hydrogenated soybean oil." *Journal of the American Oil Chemists' Society* 79, no. 8 (2002): 803–808. doi:10.1007/s11746-002-0562-y.

Saraf, S. and Kaur, C. "In vitro sun protection factor determination of herbal oils used in cosmetics." *Pharmacognosy Research* 2, no. 1 (2010): 22–25. doi:10.4103/0974-8490.60586.

Shim, C. and Williams, M. H., Jr. "Effect of odors in asthma." *American Journal of Medicine* 80, no. 1 (1986): 18–22. https://www.ncbi.nlm.nih.gov/pubmed/3079951

Stahlhut, R. W., et al. "Concentrations of urinary phthalate metabolites are associated with increased waist circumference and insulin resistance in adult U.S. males." *Environmental Health Perspectives* 115, no. 6 (Jun 2007): 876–882. doi: 10.1289/ehp.9882.

Straub, L., et al. "Neonicotinoid insecticides can serve as inadvertent insect contraceptives." *Proceedings of the Royal Society B: Biological Sciences* 283, no. 1835 (July 27, 2016). doi:10.1098/rspb.2016.0506

Thyssen, J. P., et al. "Contact sensitization to fragrances in the general population: a Koch's approach may reveal the burden of disease." *British Journal of Dermatology* 460, no. 4 (2009): 729–735. doi: 10.111/j.1365-2133.2008.09022.x

U.S. National Toxicology Program. "Carcinogenesis Studies of Methyleugenol (CAS NO. 93-15-2) in F344/N Rats and B6C3F1 Mice (Gavage Studies)." National Toxicology Program Technical Report Series 491 (Jul 2000): 1–412.

U.S. National Toxicology Program. "NTP toxicology and carcinogenesis studies of 2,4-hexadienal (89% trans,trans isomer, CAS No. 142-83-6; 11% cis,trans isomer) (Gavage Studies)." National Toxicology Program Technical Report Series 509 (2003): 1–290.

CONVERSIONS

VOLUME CONVERSIONS

U.S.	Metric
1 tablespoon / ½ fluid ounce	15 milliliters
¼ cup / 2 fluid ounces	60 milliliters
⅓ cup / 3 fluid ounces	90 milliliters
½ cup / 4 fluid ounces	120 milliliters
1 cup / 8 fluid ounces	240 milliliters

WEIGHT CONVERSIONS

U.S.	Metric
1 ounce	30 grams
⅓ pound	150 grams
1 pound	450 grams

TEMPERATURE CONVERSIONS

Fahrenheit (°F)	Celsius (°C)
140°F	60°C
150°F	65°C
160°F	70°C
350°F	175°C
375°F	190°C
400°F	200°C
425°F	220°C
450°F	230°C

INDEX

Note: Recipe names appear in upper/lower case, as in Anti-Acne Lotion.

ACKNOWLEDGMENTS

When an author writes a book, so many of the stories shared are scenes of family life. So thank you family, for giving me stories to share. Thank you Robin, Sarah, and Christopher for believing that I could write a book within the tight deadlines of this project and telling me "go for it." Robin, you gave me the time I needed to write, fielded the phone calls, and did the cooking, the dishes, and the laundry more times than I can count. Sarah, you checked up on the project weekly from Jerusalem while busy with your own heavy writing schedule. You beta-read the first draft at the last minute while I was still writing the final chapters. Your suggestions made the book stronger. Christopher, you encouraged me more than you know. Ian, I wish you were here: I5005EU.

Thank you to my friends, Kathie Lapcevic, Angi Schneider, Jessica Knowles Lane, and Tessa Zundel, for supporting me every day on social media, offering bee photos, critiquing my photographs, and sharing information and insights on writing, blogging, and marketing. One day we will meet face to face and share a pot of herbal tea together. Then I'll be able to thank you in person.

Kris Bordessa and Angela England, thank you for your input on the project. Your advice made this a stronger book and your insights helped me move from writer to author. I couldn't have written this book without you.

Connie Meyer and Angi Schneider, thank you for loaning me your beekeeping experiences and your photos for the book. Thanks for your generous spirits.

Sheryl McIver, Leana Adrian, Joyce and Elliot Teskey, many thanks for letting me use your amazing toys for photo props. Elliot, thank you for loaning me your expertise in photography.

Casie Vogel, Renee Rutledge, and the team at Ulysses Press, thank you for being so awesome to work with, for making the book beautiful and inviting, and for working with me through the editing process. Your input was invaluable in shaping the final project for the better. It was a joy to have you on my team.

Thank you to all the natural beekeepers who tirelessly put the welfare of their bees before honey harvests. May your numbers increase and your markets expand.

Thank you, Reader, for picking up this book and deciding to make a difference for yourself, for your family, and for the bees.

ABOUT THE AUTHOR

Chris Dalziel is a teacher, author, gardener, and herbalist with 30-plus years of experience growing herbs and formulating herbal remedies, skin care products, soaps, and candles. She teaches workshops and writes extensively about gardening, crafts, and medicinal herbs on her blog at JoybileeFarm.com.

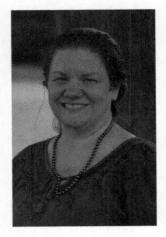

Chris is the author of the *The Beginner's Book of Essential Oils: Learning to Use Your First 10 Essential Oils with Confidence, Homegrown Healing: from Seed to Apothecary,* and this book, *The Beeswax Workshop.* She is also a contributing writer to *The Biblical Herbal E-Magazine*, the *FermenTools Blog*, and the *Attainable Sustainable* blog.

Formerly the president of the Boundary Artisan Association and the Boundary Spinners and Weavers Guild, Chris led both organizations through two successful art gallery shows. She's won awards for her textile designs and was featured in *Ashford Wheel Magazine* in 2011.

Chris lives with her husband, Robin, in the mountains of British Columbia on a 140-acre ranch, with sheep, dairy goats, llamas, and a few retired chickens. They have three adult children and three granddaughters.